Contents

Preface 4

English => Spanish 7

Reception 8
Anamnesis 14
Massage 26
Manual therapy 31
PNF 41
Mulligan 46
Exercises 49
Gait training 57
Lymphatic drainage 58
Electrotherapy 62
Pelvic floor exercises 65
Breathing therapy 70
Useful 73

English => Italian 75

Reception 76
Anamnesis 82
Massage 94
Manual therapy 99
PNF 109
Mulligan 115
Exercises 118
Gait Training 125
Lymphatic drainage 127
Electrotherapy 131
Pelvic floor exercises 134
Breathing therapy 138
Useful 141

English => French 143

Reception 144
Anamnesis 150
Massage 162
Manual therapy 167
PNF 177
Mulligan 183
Exercises 186
Gait training 194
Lymphatic drainage 196
Electrotherapy 200
Pelvic floor exercises 203
Breathing therapy 207
Useful 210

English => German 212

Reception 213
Anamnesis 219
Massage 231
Manual therapy 236
PNF 246
Mulligan 251
Exercises 254
Gait training 261
Lymphatic drainage 263
Electrotherapy 267
pelvic floor exercises 270
Breathing therapy 274
Useful 277

English => Turkish...**279**

Reception...280
Anamnesis...286
Massage...298
Manual therapy...302
PNF..312
Mulligan..317
Exercises...320
Gait training...327
Lymphatic drainage..329
Electrotherapy..333
Pelvic floor exercises..336
Breathing therapy...340
Useful...343

Thanks..345

Bibliography...346

Preface

Who am I?

My name is Caroline Braun and I created the Little Physio.
I studied translation and worked as a freelance translator.
I then decided to change my way of living and became a physiotherapist / physical therapist.
I've been working as a physical therapist for over 10 years in different hospitals as well as in private practices.

Why did I create Little Physio?

My experience has shown me the difficulties of treating patients who don't speak the same language.
It's difficult and even sometimes impossible to diagnose or treat the patient correctly.
The consequences for the patient are disastrous.

Many people think that the patient has to speak the language of the country he or she lives in.
Even if correct it's also not always possible.
Some people are not able to learn or have just arrived.
Others might be on vacation or are only here temporarily to work.

I am a physical therapist and my job is not to judge but to treat the patients.
And I have to treat them the best I can.

That's why I created "Little Physio".

This translator enables the therapist to communicate and to treat foreign patients.

Your therapy will become easier and better.

The book is divided into 14 chapters like "Reception", "Massage", "Manual therapy", "Exercises" and so on. This makes it easier and faster for you to find the sentences you need.

In addition to the book, you have the opportunity to get the **Little Physio App for mobile phones and tabs, iphone and ipad.**

The Apps are available on the Apple Appstore and on the Googleplaystore.

The **Little Physio Apps are the audio version of the books.**

It is as easy as clicking on the needed sentence and your cell phone or tab "speaks" it out in the foreign language.

You can see a demo on:

littlephysio.com

or on

youtube

I became a physical therapist to help others, no matter if they speak my language or not.

Now, it is possible!

English => Spanish

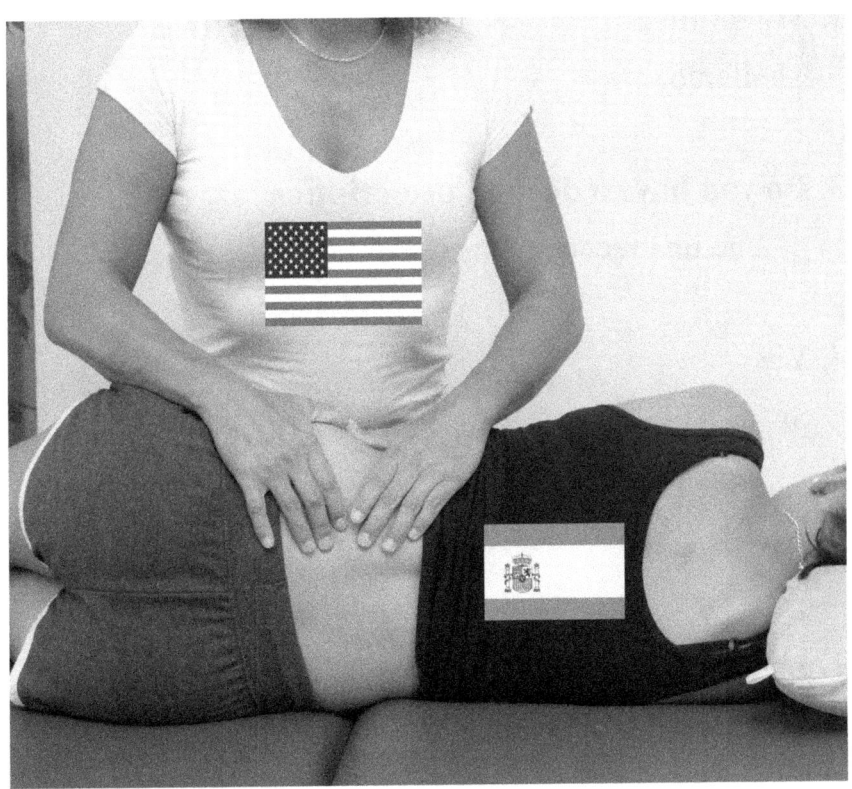

Reception

El recibimiento

1. Hello

Buenos días

2. My name is

Me llamo...

3. Do you have a doctor's prescription?

¿Tiene una receta médica?

4. Yes

Sí

5. No

No

6. Do you have your insurance card?

¿Tiene su tarjeta de seguro social?

7. **Would you please bring the insurance card next time?**

   ¿Puede traer su tarjeta de seguro social la próxima vez?

8. **Would you please write down your phone number?**

   ¿Me podría apuntar su número de teléfono, por favor?

9. **There is a mistake in the prescription. You have to go back to your doctor and have him issue a new one.**

   En la receta hay un error, usted debe ir de nuevo al médico para que le dé una receta nueva.

10. **Do you have a report / X-ray / CT- images from your doctor?**

    ¿Le ha dado su médico un informe médico, radiografías o exploraciones TAC (Tomografía axial computarizada)?

11. **Would you please bring the x-rays / the report with you next time?**

    ¿Podría traer la próxima vez el informe y las imágenes médicas, o sea, las radiografías y tomografías?

12. Here are your appointments

Aquí tiene sus citas.

13. If these appointments don't work for you, please let me know.

En caso de que no le vengan bien las citas, me lo dice.

14. This one doesn't work?

¿Esa fecha no le viene bien?

15. Not on this day at all?

¿Tampoco ese día no le viene bien?

16. Rather in the morning?

¿Le conviene mejor por la mañana?

17. Rather in the afternoon?

¿Le conviene mejor por la tarde?

18. Monday

El lunes

19. Tuesday

El martes

20. Wednesday
El miércoles

21. Thursday
El jueves

22. Friday
El viernes

23. Saturday
El sábado

24. Sunday
El domingo

25. I'm sorry, you are too early
Lo siento mucho, pero usted ha venido muy temprano.

26. I'm sorry you, are too late
Lo siento mucho, pero usted ha venido muy tarde.

27. This week won't work
Esta semana no me viene bien.

28. Today doesn't work
Hoy no me viene bien.

29. Not before next week
Sólo puede ser a partir de la semana próxima.

30. Not before next month
Puede ser sólo a partir del próximo mes.

31. The therapist is on vacation
Su terapeuta está de vacaciones

32. The therapist is ill
Su terapeuta está enferma / enfermo

33. Would you like to work with a different therapist?
¿Desea cambiar de terapeuta?

34. Yes
Si

35. No
No

36. Would you like to continue with the same therapist?

¿Quiere quedarse con su mismo/a terapeuta?

37. Would you rather wait until your therapist is back?

¿Quiere esperar hasta que regrese su terapeuta?

38. Here is your bill.

Aquí tiene su factura.

39. Would you like to pay now?

¿Desea abonar ahora?

40. Do you want to pay cash?

¿Desea pagar en efectivo?

Anamnesis

Anamnesis

1. Please undress
¿ Puede quitarse la ropa, por favor?

2. Can you please take off your top ?
¿Puede dejar libre la parte de arriba?

3. Can you please take off your pants?
¿Puede quitarse los pantalones?

4. Can you please take off your skirt?
¿Puede quitarse la falda?

5. Are you in pain?
¿Siente dolor?

6. Yes
Sí

7. No

No

8. Show me where it hurts

Muéstreme por favor dónde le duele

9. Where does it hurt?

¿Dónde siente dolor?

10. Is the pain radiating into your arm?

¿El dolor se inicia en el brazo?

11. Is the pain radiating into your leg?

¿El dolor se inicia en la pierna?

12. Where does the pain radiate into?

¿Hacia dónde se dispersan los dolores?

13. Show me

Me lo muestra, por favor

14. Do you feel numbness?

¿Siente una sensación de adormecimiento?

15. Where?

¿Dónde?

16. Do you have paralytic symptoms?

¿Tiene síntomas de entumecimiento?

17. Do you feel formication?

¿Tiene sensación de hormigueo?

18. Where?

¿Dónde?

19. When did it start?

¿Desde cuándo siente esos síntomas?

20. For days

Desde hace días

21. For weeks

Desde hace semanas

22. For months

Desde hace meses

23. For years

Desde hace años

24. What does the pain feel like?

¿Cómo es el dolor?

25. Acute

Es un dolor agudo

26. Dull

Es un dolor sordo

27. Dragging

Siente tirones

28. Did the pain develop slowly?

¿El dolor se ha iniciado lentamente?

29. Did the pain develop fast?

¿El dolor comenzó repentinamente?

30. Does the pain last for a long time?

¿El dolor es persistente?

31. Several seconds

Por varios segundos

32. Several minutes

Durante varios minutos

33. Several hours

Durante varias horas

34. Several days

Durante varios días

35. Did you have an accident?

¿Tuvo un accidente?

36. Have you had treatment yet?

¿Ya le han tratado?

37. Yes

Sí

38. No

No

39. Do you have high blood pressure?

¿Tiene hipertensión arterial?

40. Do you have diabetes?

¿Tiene diabetes?

41. Are you dizzy?

¿Se marea?

42. Are you pregnant?

¿Está embarazada?

43. What month?

¿En qué mes de embarazo está?

44. Do you take pain killers?

¿Toma analgésicos?

45. Do you take blood thinning medication?

¿Toma medicamentos anticoagulantes u otro tipo de medicamento?

46. Do you have problems with your thyroid?

¿Tiene problemas de tiroides?

47. Do you have heart problems?

¿Tiene problemas del corazón?

48. Do you have a headache?

¿Tiene dolores de cabeza?

49. Did you have surgery?

¿Se ha sometido a una operación quirúrgica?

50. When did you have surgery?

¿Cuándo fue la operación?

51. A few days ago

Hace días

52. A few months ago

Hace meses

53. A few years ago

Hace años

54. You have to see a doctor.

Usted tiene que ir al médico

55. Does it hurt when you are moving?

¿Siente dolores por el peso?

56. Do you have pain while resting?

¿Sufre de artrosis?

57. When does it hurt most? When is the pain worst?

¿Cuándo siente esos dolores intensamente?

58. In the morning

Por la mañana

59. In the evening

Por la tarde

60. At night

Por la noche

61. Always the same

Continuamente

62. While going up

Al caminar cuesta arriba

63. While going down

Al caminar cuesta abajo

64. Going up the stairs

Al subir las escaleras

65. Going down the stairs

Al bajar las escaleras

66. While sitting for a long time

¿Al estar sentado durante largo tiempo?

67. After sitting for a long time

¿Después de haber estado sentado por largo tiempo?

68. While doing small movements?

¿Al hacer pequeños movimientos?

69. Were you in the hospital / in rehab?

¿Estuvo en un hospital o en un tratamiento médico?

70. For how long?

¿Por cuánto tiempo?

71. Several days

Durante varios días

72. Several weeks

Durante varias semanas

73. Several months

Durante varios meses

74. When did you get discharged from the hospital?

¿Cuándo le dieron de alta del hospital?

75. Yesterday

Ayer

76. The day before yesterday

Antes de ayer

77. A few days ago
   Hace un par de días

78. How many?
   ¿Cuánto?

79. A few weeks ago
   Hace un par de semanas

80. A few months ago
   Hace un par de meses

Massage

Masajes

1. Please get undressed
¿ Puede quitarse la ropa, por favor?

2. Can you please take off your top?
¿Puede dejar libre la parte de arriba?

3. Can you please take off your pants?
¿Puede quitarse los pantalones?

4. Can you please take off your skirt?
¿Puede quitarse la falda?

5. Lie down on your back
Póngase boca arriba, por favor

6. Lie down on your stomach
Póngase boca abajo, por favor

7. Lie down on your right side

Recuéstese sobre el costado derecho, por favor

8. Lie down on your left side

Recuéstese sobre el costado izquierdo, por favor

9. This is for your head

Ponga la cabeza aquí, por favor

10. Would you like a blanket?

¿Quiere una manta?`

11. Are you cold?

¿Le hace frío?

12. Are you too warm?

¿Le hace calor?

13. Put your right arm down

Coloque el brazo derecho hacia abajo

14. Put your right arm next to your head
   Coloque el brazo derecho hacia arriba

15. Align your right arm alongside your body
   Coloque el brazo derecho junto a su cuerpo

16. Put your left arm down
   Coloque el brazo izquierdo hacia abajo

17. Put your left arm next to your head
   Coloque el brazo izquierdo hacia arriba

18. Align your left arm alongside your body
   Coloque el brazo izquierdo junto a su cuerpo

19. Sit down please.
   Tome asiento, por favor

20. Relax your shoulders
   Afloje los hombros

21. Please look straigt ahead

Mire hacia adelante

22. Does it hurt?

¿Duele?

23. Do I hurt you?

¿Le causo dolor?

24. Show me where it hurts.

Múestreme dónde le duele

25. Is the pressure ok?

¿Está bien la presión?

26. Yes?

¿Sí?

27. No?

¿No?

28. Harder?

¿Presiono mas fuerte?

29. Softer?

¿Menos presión?

30. Better?

¿Está mejor así?

31. Worse?

¿Está peor así?

Manual therapy

Terapia manual

1. Please get undressed
 ¿ Puede quitarse la ropa, por favor?

2. Can you please take off your top?
 ¿Puede dejar libre la parte de arriba?

3. Can you please take off your pants?
 ¿Puede quitarse los pantalones?

4. Can you please take off your skirt?
 ¿Puede quitarse la falda?

5. Where does it hurt?
 ¿Dónde siente dolor?

6. Has it improved since the last treatment?
 ¿Ha mejorado el dolor desde el último tratamiento?

7. Has it gotten worse?

¿Ha empeorado el dolor?

8. Has the pain increased?

¿Siente ahora más dolores?

9. Has the pain gotten less?

¿Siente ahora menos dolores?

10. Where does it hurt now?

¿Dónde siente ahora los dolores?

11. Stand on one leg please.

Quédese de pie sobre una pierna

12. Please stand on the other leg now.

Ahora quédese de pie sobre la otra pierna

13. Stand on your heels

Quédese de pie sobre sus talones

14. Stand on your tiptoes

Quédese de pie sobre la punta de sus pies

15. Sit down please

Siéntese por favor

16. Round your back

Inclínise hacia abajo la parte superior del cuerpo

17. Put your chin to your chest

Incline su cabeza hacia abajo

18. Does it pull?

¿Le tira?

19. Is it painful?

¿Es doloroso?

20. Is the pain less now?

¿Ahora le duele menos?

21. Is the pain worse now?

¿Y así le duele más?

22. Better?

¿Está mejor así?

23. Worse?

¿Está peor así?

24. Put your head back

Levante la cabeza, por favor

25. Lift your head up, look up

Mantenga la cabeza arriba / Mire hacia arriba

26. Put your head down, look down

Mantenga la cabeza abajo / Mire hacia abajo

27. Turn your head to the left

Gire la cabeza hacia la izquierda

28. Turn your head to the right

Gire la cabeza hacia la derecha

29. Tilt your head to the left

Incline la cabeza hacia la izquierda

30. Tilt your head to the right

Incline la cabeza hacia la derecha

31. Relax
Póngase más flojo

32. Do not help. I will do the movements, you relax
No ayude, yo haré el movimiento, usted se relaja

33. Put your arms up
Levante los brazos

34. Put your right arm up
Levante el brazo derecho

35. Put your right arm down
Baje el brazo derecho

36. Put your left arm up
Levante el brazo izquierdo

37. Put your left arm down
Baje el brazo izquierdo

38. Bend your leg
Flexione la pierna

39. Extend your leg

Estire la pierna

40. Bend your knee

Doble la rodilla

41. Extend your knee

Estire la rodilla

42. Lift your leg

Levante la pierna

43. Lie on your back

Póngase boca arriba

44. Lie on your stomach

Póngase boca abajo

45. Lie on your right side

Póngase sobre el costado derecho

46. Lie on your left side

Póngase sobre el costado izquierdo

47. Put your head here, please
  Ponga la cabeza aquí, por favor

48. Sit down
  Tome asiento por favor

49. Please participate with ease
  Siga haciendo el movimiento levemente

50. Press against my resistance
  Presione en contra de mi resistencia

51. Press harder
  Presione con más fuerza

52. Press not so hard
  Presione levemente

53. This is an exercise to do at home
  Éste es un ejercicio para hacerlo en casa

54. Bend your legs and pull your knees to your thighs
  Ponga los pies debajo de las rodillas

55. Tighten your Abdomen
Ponga tenso el vientre

56. Squeeze your buttocks
Ponga tenso el trasero

57. Tense your legs
Ponga tensas las piernas

58. Tense your arms
Ponga tensos los brazos

59. Relax
Relájese

60. It might hurt a little
Puede ser que le duela un poco

61. I will show you first, then you repeat
Le muestro el ejercicio, y después usted lo repite

62. Do 3 sets with 10 repetitions
Realice tres series de 10 repeticiones

63. Do 3 sets with 15 repetitions

Realice tres series de 15 repeticiones

64. Do 3 sets with 20 repetitions

Realice tres series de 20 repeticiones

65. Do 3 sets with 30 repetitions

Realice tres series de 30 repeticiones

66. Once a week

Una vez por semana

67. Twice a week

Dos veces por semana

68. Three times a week

Tres veces por semana

69. Once a day

Una vez por día

70. Twice a day

Dos veces por día

71. Three times a day

Tres veces por día

72. Do the exercise in front of a mirror

Realice el ejercicio delante del espejo

73. Sit down in front of a mirror

Siéntese delante del espejo

74. Stand in front of a mirror

Póngase de pie delante del espejo

75. It is not supposed to hurt

No tiene que sentir dolor

76. This is not supposed to happen

Eso no puede pasar

PNF

FNP (Facilitación Neuromuscular proprioceptiva)

1. **Lie on your back**
   Póngase boca arriba

2. **Lie on your stomach**
   Póngase boca abajo

3. **Lie on your right side**
   Póngase sobre el costado derecho

4. **Lie on your left side**
   Póngase sobre el costado izquierdo

5. **Put your head here, please**
   Ponga la cabeza aquí, por favor

6. **I will show you what the movement should look like**
   Le muestro cómo tiene que ser el movimiento

7. I will do the movement, relax your arm
   Yo haré el movimiento y usted suelte el brazo

8. I will do the movement, relax your leg
   Yo haré el movimiento y usted afloje la pierna

9. Press against my resistance now
   Ahora presione en contra de mi resistencia

10. Open your hand and extend your fingers
   Abra la mano y los dedos, por favor

11. Close your hand aroung mine
   Cierre la mano y los dedos, por favor

12. Extend your arm
   Estire el brazo y el codo, por favor

13. Bend your elbow
   Doble el brazo

14. Put your leg up
   Levante la pierna

15. Put your leg down
 Baje la pierna

16. Tense your leg in this direction
 Ponga tensa la pierna hacia esta dirección

17. Bend your knee
 Doble la rodilla

18. Extend your knee
 Estire la rodilla

19. Bend your hips
 Flexione la cadera

20. Extend your hips
 Estire la cadera

21. Relax
 Relajar / aflojar

22. More
 Más

23. Less

Menos

24. Harder

Con más intensidad

25. Softer

Levemente

26. Slower

Lentamente

27. Faster

Más rápido

28. Press upward

Presione hacia arriba

29. Press downward

Presione hacia abajo

30. Now in the other direction

Ahora presione en otra dirección

31. Towards your opposite shoulder
   Presione en dirección al hombro contrario

32. Towards your opposite hip
   Presione en dirección a la cadera contraria

33. Towards the ear
   En dirección a su oreja

34. Towards the nose
   En dirección a su nariz

35. Towards the window
   En dirección a la ventana

36. Towards the door
   En dirección a la puerta

37. Towards the wall
   En dirección a la pared

38. Towards the clock
   En dirección al reloj

Mulligan

Mulligan

1. Show me which movement causes the pain
Muéstreme con qué movimiento siente dolor

2. Relax
Relájese

3. Repeat the movement once more
Ahora realice el movimiento de nuevo

4. Is it better?
¿Es mejor así?

5. Do you have pain going upstairs?
¿Siente dolor al subir las escaleras?

6. Do you have pain going downstairs?

¿Siente dolor al bajar las escaleras?

7. Is it better like this?

¿Es mejor así?

8. You are not supposed to be in pain. Please say Stop if it hurts

No debe sentir dolor, en caso de que sienta dolor me dice: "Pare".

9. If the strap hurts, I can put a pad between you and the strap

Si el cinturón le provoca dolor, coloco un almohadón entre el cinturón y usted.

10. You can do this exercise with a towel at home

En casa puede hacer el ejercicio con una toalla

11. you can do this exercise at home with an elastic band

En casa puede hacer el ejercicio con una cinta Thera-Band (cinta elástica de látex)

12. You can do this exercise at home with a stick

En casa puede hacer el ejercicio con una vara o bastón

13. The ball can be purchased at a sporting goods store

La pelota la puede comprar en una tienda de artículos de deportes

14. The elastic band can be purchased at a sporting goods store

La cinta Thera-Band la puede comprar en una tienda de artículos de deportes.

15. It should be red

Debe ser roja

16. It should be green

Debe ser verde

Exercises

Ejercicios

1. Bend
Flexionar

2. Extend
Estirarse

3. Flex
Tensionar

4. Relax
Relajarse

5. Move your buttocks backwards
Ponga el trasero hacia atrás

6. tense your abdomen / do not relax
Ponga tenso el vientre / déjelo tenso

7. Remain like this for a few seconds, then relax

Permanezca así durante algunos segundos y luego afloje

8. Do not move

No debe hacer ningún movimiento

9. This is for your coordination

Esto ayuda a la coordinación

10. Do 3 sets with 10 repetitions

Haga tres Series de 10 repeticiones

11. Do 3 sets with 15 repetitions

Haga tres Series de 15 repeticiones

12. Do 3 sets with 20 repetitions

Haga tres Series de 20 repeticiones

13. Do 3 sets with 30 repetitions

Haga tres Series de 30 repeticiones

14. Take a break between the sets

Incluya periodos de descanso entre los ejercicios

15. A few seconds

Un periodo de descanso por algunos segundos

16. A few minutes

Un periodo de descanso por algunos minutos

17. How many

¿Cuántas veces hay que practicar?

18. Once a week

Una vez por semana

19. Twice a week

Dos veces por semana

20. Three times a week

Tres veces por semana

21. Once a day

Una vez por día

22. Twice a day

Dos veces por día

23. Three times a day

Tres veces por día

24. Do the exercise while standing in front of a mirror

Haga los ejercicios delante del espejo

25. Sit in front of the mirror

Siéntese delante del espejo

26. Stand in front of the mirror

Póngase de pie delante del espejo

27. This is for strengthening

Esto sirve para el fortalecimiento

28. Do it at home every day

Practique los ejercicios todos los días en casa

29. Do the exercises in front of the mirror so that you can correct yourself

Haga los ejercicios delante del espejo para que los pueda corregir.

30. This is not supposed to happen
   Eso no puede pasar

31. This is wrong
   Eso está mal

32. This is correct
   Eso está bien

33. Slow
   Lentamente

34. Slower
   Más lento

35. Fast
   Rápido

36. Faster
   Más rápido

37. don't jerk
   Que no sea de golpe

38. Your are not supposed to be in pain during the exercise

No debe sentir ningún dolor al hacer los ejercicios

39. If you are in pain doing the exercise please stop and tell me next time you are here.

Si siente dolor al hacer los ejercicios, déjelos, no continúe con ellos y me lo dice la próxima vez.

40. Did you do the exercises?

¿Practicó los ejercicios?

41. Did you feel any pain?

¿Sintió dolor al hacer los ejercicios?

42. Show me where it hurt?

Muéstreme dónde sintió dolores

43. Show me how you do the exercises?

Muéstreme cómo hizo los ejercicios

44. Stand on your right leg

Quédese de pie sobre la pierna derecha

45. Stand on your left leg

Quédese de pie sobre la pierna izquierda

46. Stand on one leg

Manténgase sobre una sola pierna

47. This is for balance

Esto sirve para el equilibrio

48. Try not to move

Intente no tambalear

49. Try to include this exercise in your daily routine

Este movimiento lo puede incorporar en sus tareas diarias.

Gait training

Reeducación de los patrones de la marcha

1. Stand straight
Póngase de pie con la espalda recta

2. Take smaller steps
Haga pequeños pasos

3. Take bigger steps
Dé pasos más grandes

4. Take regular steps
Dé pasos regulares o normales

5. Roll your foot from heel to toe
Haga girar el pie hacia ambos lados

6. First on your heel, roll your foot, then press your foot forward to your toes

Primero aciente el pie sobre los talones y luego hágalo girar hacia ambos lados y después presione el pie hacia adelante con el talón.

7. The crutch goes on the same side as your injured leg

La muleta (o bastón inglés) es el apoyo de la pierna enferma, por lo tanto deben ir juntos.

8. Swing your arms loosely by your body

Mueva relajadamente los brazos de un lado a otro junto a su cuerpo.

Lymphatic drainage

Drenaje linfático

1. **The blood pressure cannot be taken on this arm nor can blood be drawn**

   En este brazo no se puede medir la presión ni poner una inyección.

2. **Preferably you should not get hurt**

   Debe evitar no lastimarse

3. **You are not allowed to take a hot bath or lie in the sun for too long**

   Usted no debe tomar un baño con agua caliente ni estar en sol durante mucho tiempo.

4. **If you have a painful rash, see a doctor immediately**

   En caso de que tenga una erupción cutánea dolorosa debe asistir de inmediato al médico.

5. Put your legs up multiple times per day

Varias veces al día coloque las piernas hacia arriba.

6. Put your leg up several times a day

Varias veces al día coloque la pierna hacia arriba.

7. Put your arm up multiple times a day

Varias veces al día coloque el brazo hacia arriba.

8. Do you have a surgical stocking?

¿Tiene una media de compresión?

9. Do you have surgical stockings?

¿Tiene medias de compresión?

10. You have to wear the stocking every day

Tiene que llevar la media todos los días.

11. You have to wear the stockings every day

Tiene que llevar las medias todos los días

12. You have to wear the stocking night and day

La media la tiene que llevar día y noche

13. You have to wear the stockings night and day

Las medias las tiene que llevar día y noche.

14. You shouldn't wear tight-fitting clothes

No debe ponerse ropa estrecha

15. Lie on your back

Póngase boca arriba

16. Lie on your stomach

Póngase boca abajo

17. Can you lie on your stomach or would your rather sit?

¿Puede ponerse boca abajo o prefiere estar sentado?

18. Sit?

¿Quiere estar sentado?

19. Put one leg up

Ponga el pie debajo de la rodilla

20. Put both legs up

Ponga los pies debajo de las rodillas

21. Slide a little towards me

Córrase un poco hacia mí, por favor

22. Slide to the left

Córrase hacia la izquierda

23. Slide to the right

Córrase hacia la derecha

24. Slide up

Córrase hacia arriba en dirección a su cabeza

25. Slide down

Córrase hacia abajo en dirección a sus pies

26. Does it hurt?

¿Le duele?

27. It shouldn't hurt

No debe sentir ningún dolor

Electrotherapy

Terapia eléctrica

1. I will attach 2 electrodes

Le voy a colocar dos electrodos

2. I will attach 4 electrodes

Le voy a colocar cuatro electrodos

3. There is no electricity yet

Todavía no pasa la electricidad

4. I will increase the electricity slowly

Lentamente voy a ir subiendo la electricidad

5. Tell me, as soon as you feel the electricity

Dígame por favor, cuando empiece a sentir la electricidad

6. Do you feel the electricity?

¿Siente la electricidad?

7. It should be comfortable

Tiene que ser agradable

8. Is it comfortable?

¿Es agradable?

9. You should feel the electricity only slightly

Usted debe sentir la electricidad sólo muy leve.

10. I will turn down the electricity until you can't feel it anymore

Ahora voy a bajar la electricidad hasta que usted no la sienta más.

11. It will take about 10 minutes

Va a durar aproximadamente unos diez minutos

12. It will take about 15 minutes

Va a durar aproximadamente unos quince minutos

13. It will take about 20 minutes

Va a durar aproximadamente unos veinte minutos

14. I will take off the electrodes once it is finished

Cuando haya terminado, vendré y le quitaré los electrodos

15. If you have a problem, call me

Si tiene algún problema, me llama

16. I will be next-door

Yo estoy a lado

Pelvic floor exercises

Ejercicios para el suelo pélvico o periné

<u>Short</u>

1. **The pelvic floor is the muscle between your pubic bone and your tailbone**

   El suelo pélvico es el conjunto de músculos que se extiende desde el hueso púbico en la parte frontal hasta el hueso de la cola (cóxis) en la parte posterior.

2. **Its function is mainly to close the openings there**

   La función del suelo pélvico es principalmente cerrar todos los orificios que se encuentran en la zona pélvica.

3. **It works together with you abdominal muscles and your diaphragm**

   El suelo pélvico hace un trabajo en conjunto con la musculatura abdominal y con el diafragma.

4. In order to strengthen your pelvic floor you have to use these muscles as well

Por lo tanto hay que hacer trabajar a esa musculatura para fortalecer el suelo pélvico.

5. Try to tense your pelvic floor, acting like have to use the bathroom but you can't go

Intente apretar los músculos principales que se extienden a lo largo del suelo pélvico y esto lo hará de la siguiente manera: Haga como si tuviera muchas ganas de ir al baño, pero reténgalas.

Long

1. **The pelvic floor is the muscle between ischial tuberosities, pubic and tailbone**

   El suelo pélvico es el músculo ubicado entre el esquión derecho e izquierdo, el coxis(el hueso en que remata la columna vertebral) y el pubis.

2. **The pelvic floor helps to control the function of urinating and bowel movement. With regular training you can prevent incontinence or lessen exiting problems**

   El suelo pélvico contribuye esencialmente al control de la salida de orina y materia fecal. A través del ejercicio diario puede prevenir la salida involuntaria de orina y materia fecal o influir favorablemente en otros problemas de la misma índole.

3. **In addition, the pelvic floor holds and supports the organs in your abdomen. Thats why regular pelvic floor training works against prolapse problems**

   Además el suelo de la pelvis es el apoyo de los órganos abdominales ya que éste los sostiene desde abajo. Por eso usted pude ayudar a prevenir los problemas de control de vejiga al ejercitar los músculos del suelo pélvico.

4. To fulfill these functions, the pelvic floor works with the abdominal muscles and the diaphragm, which is the most important respiratory muscle.

Para poder lograr ese objetivo, los músculos del suelo pélvico realizan su trabajo junto con la musculatura abdominal y el diafragma. El diafragma es un músculo muy importante para la respiración.

5. In order to strengthen your pelvic floor you have to use these muscles as well

Por esta razón hay que hacer trabajar a estos músculos para fortalecer el suelo pélvico.

6. Try to tighten your pelvic floor, imagining closing your vagina and anus

Intente contraer los músculos del suelo pélvico y lo hará de la siguiente manera: Imaginese que está cerrando el ano y su vagina.

7. Try to tighten your pelvic floor, acting like have to use the toilet ▯but you can't go

Intente contraer los músculos del suelo pélvico y lo hará de la siguiente manera: Haga como si tuviera muchas ganas de ir al baño, pero reténgalas

8. Inhale deeply. Exhale slowly tensing your abdominal muscles

Respire profundamente, contraiga el abdomen al expulsar el aire lentamente.

9. I will show you, and then you do it

Yo le mostraré el ejercicio primero y luego usted lo repetirá.

Breathing therapy

Terapia respiratoria

1. Inhale through your nose

Respire por la nariz

2. Exhale through your mouth

Espire el aire por la boca.

3. I will show you, and then you do it

Yo haré primero el ejercicio y después usted lo repetirá.

4. Slowly

Lento

5. Slower

Más lento

6. Fast

Rápido

7. Faster
Más rápido

8. Deeply
Profundo

9. Deeper
Más profundo

10. Casual
Ligero

11. More casually
Más ligero

12. Inhale more into your abdomen
Inspire el aire por su nariz hacia la parte baja del vientre

13. Your abdomen should expand when inhaling
El vientre debe inflarse a través de la inspiración

14. Put your hands on your abdomen

Coloque las manos sobre su vientre.

15. Put your hands on your ribcage

Coloque sus manos sobre el tórax.

16. Your hands should be moving on your abdomen when inhaling

Inspire de modo que el aire mueva el vientre y sus manos.

Useful

Frases útiles

1. Hello
Buenos días / Buenas tardes

2. Goodbye
Adiós

3. Please
Por favor

4. Thank you
Gracias

5. Relax
Aflojar

6. Does it hurt?
¿Duele?

7. Is it better now?

¿Está mejor así?

8. Harder?

¿Más fuerte?

9. Yes

Si

10. No

No

11. I'm sorry, I can't understand you

Lo siento, no entiendo

English => Italian

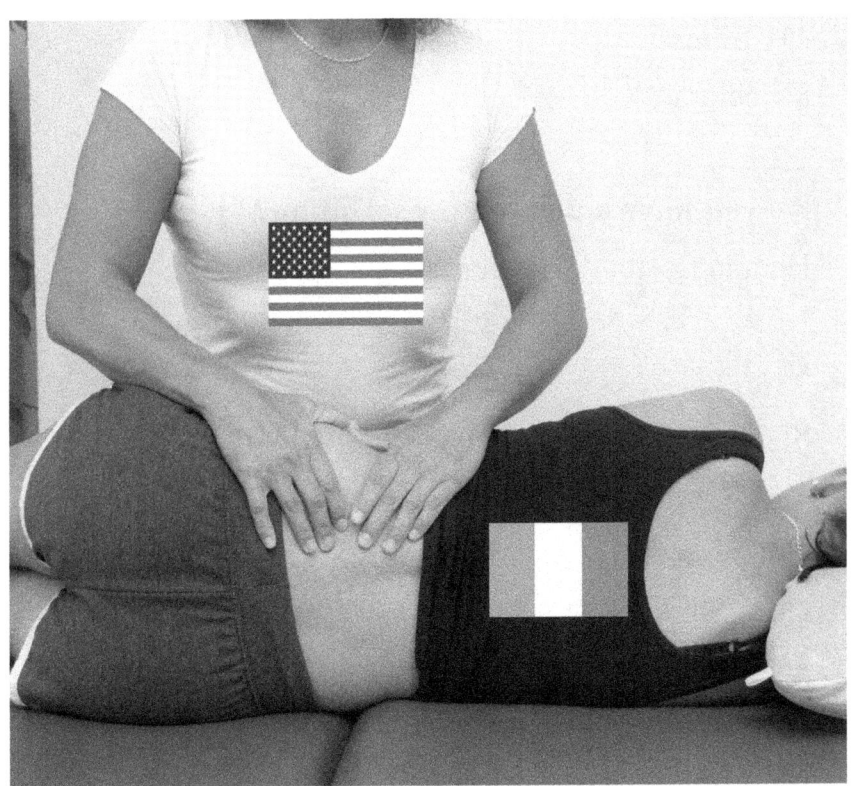

Reception

Accoglienza

1. Hello
Buon giorno

2. My name is
Mi chiamo

3. Do you have a doctor's prescription?
Ha una ricetta del dottore?

4. Yes
Si

5. No
No

6. Do you have your insurance card?
Ha il libretto assicurativo?

7. **Would you please bring the insurance card next time?**

Lo può portare la prossima volta?

8. **Would you please write down your phone number?**

Mi scrive il suo numero di telefono per favore?

9. **There is a mistake in the prescription. You have to go back to your doctor and have him issue a new one.**

Qui c´é un sbaglio sulla ricetta per piacere vada di nuovo dal dottore, a chiedergli una ricetta nuova.

10. **Do you have a report / X-ray / CT- images from your doctor?**

Ha un rapporto / Radiografia, TAC del dottore?

11. **Would you please bring the x-rays / the report with you next time?**

La prossima volta mi porti il rapporto, le radiografie?

12. **Here are your appointments**

Questi sono i suoi appuntamenti

13. If these appointments can't work for you, please let me know.

Se li appuntamenti non vanno bene per lei, melo dica.

14. This one doesn't work?

Qui non vá?

15. Not on this day at all?

Questo giorno non vá?

16. Rather in the morning?

Meglio di mattina?

17. Rather in the afternoon?

Meglio di pomeriggio?

18. Monday

Lunedì

19. Tuesday

Martedì

20. Wednesday
Mercoledì

21. Thursday
Giovedì

22. Friday
Venerdì

23. Saturday
Sabato

24. Sunday
Domenica

25. I'm sorry, you are too early
Mi dispiace, ma lei è in anticipo

26. I'm sorry, you are too late
Mi dispiace, ma lei è in ritardo

27. This week won't work
Questa settimana non vá

28. Today doesn't work
Oggi non vá

29. Not before next week
La prossima settimana

30. Not before next month
Il prossimo mese

31. The therapist is on vacation
Il terapista é in vacanze

32. The therapist is ill
Il terapista é malato

33. Would you like to work with a different therapist?
Vuole andare da un altro terapista?

34. Yes

Si

35. No

No

36. Would you like to continue with the same therapist?

Desidera lo stesso terapista?

37. Would you rather wait until your therapist is back?

Vuole aspettare finché arriva il terapista?

38. Here is your bill.

Qui é il suo conto

39. Would you like to pay now?

Vuole pagare adesso?

40. Do you want to pay cash?

Vuole pagare in contanti?

Anamnesis

Anamnesi

1. Please undress
Si spogli per favore

2. Can you please take off your top ?
Può togliersi il disopra?

3. Can you please take off your pants?
Può togliersi il pantalone?

4. Can you please take off your skirt?
Può togliersi la gonna?

5. Are you in pain?
Ha dei dolori?

6. Yes
Si

7. No
No

8. Show me where it hurts
Mi faccia vedere dove ha dolori

9. Where does it hurt?
Dove ha dolori?

10. Is the pain radiating into your arm?
Vanno per il braccio?

11. Is the pain radiating into your leg?
Vanno nella gamba?

12. Where does the pain radiate into?
Fino dove arrivanno i dolori?

13. Show me
Mi faccia vedere

14. Do you feel numbness?

Sente la mancanza di sensibilità?

15. Where?

Dove?

16. Do you have paralytic symptoms?

Ha dei sindromi di paralizzo?

17. Do you feel formication?

Ha dei formicolii?

18. Where?

Dove?

19. When did it start?

Da quando?

20. For days

Da giorni

21. For weeks

Da settimane

22. For months

Da mesi

23. For years

Da anni

24. What does the pain feel like?

Com´é il dolore?

25. Acute

Punge

26. Dull

Cupo

27. Dragging

Tira

28. Did the pain develop slowly?
Il dolore si è sviluppato piano

29. Did the pain develop fast?
Il dolore si è sviluppato subito?

30. Does the pain last for a long time?
Il dolore tiene a lungo?

31. Several seconds
Dei secondi

32. Several minutes
Dei minuti

33. Several hours
Delle ore

34. Several days
Dei giorni

35. Did you have an accident?
Ha avuto un incidente?

36. Have you had treatment yet?
È stato visitato già?

37. Yes
Si

38. No
No

39. Do you have high blood pressure?
Lei soffre di ipertensione

40. Do you have diabetes?
Ha il diabete?

41. Are you dizzy?
Soffre di vertigini?

42. Are you pregnant?
   Lei è incinta?

43. What month?
   Di quanti mesi?

44. Do you take pain killers?
   Prende dei antidolorifici?

45. Do you take blood thinning medication?
   Lei si prende dei medicamenti per diluire il sangue?

46. Do you have problems with your thyroid?
   Ha dei problemi con la tiroide?

47. Do you have heart problems?
   Ha dei problemi con il cuore?

48. Do you have a headache?
   Ha dei dolori di testa?

49. Did you have surgery?

È stato operato?

50. When did you have surgery?

Quando é stata l'operazione?

51. A few days ago

Da giorni

52. A few months ago

Da mesi

53. A few years ago

Da anni

54. You have to see a doctor.

Lei ha bisogno di andare dal dottore

55. Does it hurt when you are moving?

Ha dei dolori nel momento di sforzo?

56. Do you have pain while resting?

Ha dei dolori nel momento di riposo?

57. When does it hurt most? When is the pain worst?

In quale situazioni sono piú forte i dolori?

58. In the morning

La mattina

59. In the evening

La sera

60. At night

La notte

61. Always the same

Sempre uguale

62. While going up

Quando sale

63. While going down

Quando scende

64. Going up the stairs

Quando sale le scale

65. Going down the stairs

Quando scende le scale

66. While sitting for a long time

Mentre è seduta alungo?

67. After sitting for a long time

Dopo che è stato seduto molto tempo?

68. While doing small movements?

Mentre dei muovimenti piccoli?

69. Were you in the hospital / in rehab?

E stato all' ospedale, in casa di cura?

70. For how long?
Per quando tempo?

71. Several days
Alcuni giorni

72. Several weeks
Alcune settimane

73. Several months
Alcuni mesi

74. When did you get discharged from the hospital?
Quando è stato dimesso dall'ospedale?

75. Yesterday
Ieri

76. The day before yesterday
Avanti ieri

77. A few days ago
Un paio di giorni fa

78. How many?
Quanti?

79. A few weeks ago
Alcune settimane fa

80. A few months ago
Alcuni mesi fa

Massage

Massaggio

1. Please get undressed
Si spogli per favore

2. Can you please take off your top?
Puo togliersi il disopra?

3. Can you please take off your pants?
Puo togliersi il pantalone?

4. Can you please take off your skirt?
Puo togliersi la gonna?

5. Lie down on your back
Si puo sdraiarsi sulla schiena

6. Lie down on your stomach
Si puo sdraiarsi sulla pancia

7. Lie down on your right side

Si puo sdraiarsi sul´lato destro

8. Lie down on your left side

Si puo sdraiarsi sul´lato sinistro

9. This is for your head

La testa qui per favore

10. Would you like a blanket?

Vuole una coperta?

11. Are you cold?

Ha freddo?

12. Are you too warm?

Ha caldo?

13. Put your right arm down

Appoggi il braccio destro, sotto

14. Put your right arm next to your head

Appoggi il braccio destro, sopra

15. Align your right arm alongside your body

Appoggi il braccio destro verso il corpo

16. Put your left arm down

Appoggi il braccio sinistro, sotto

17. Put your left arm next to your head

Appoggi il braccio sinistro, sopra

18. Align your left arm alongside your body

Appoggi il braccio sinistro verso il corpo

19. Sit down please.

Si sieda per favore

20. Relax your shoulders

Lasci sciolte la spalla

21. Please look straigt ahead

Guardi avanti

22. Does it hurt?

Le fà male?

23. Do I hurt you?

Le faccio male?

24. Show me where it hurts.

Mi faccia vedere dove le fà male

25. Is the pressure ok?

Va bene la pressione cosi?

26. Yes?

SI?

27. No?

NO?

28. Harder?
Piu forte?

29. Softer?
Piu piano?

30. Better?
Meglio?

31. Worse?
Peggio?

Manual therapy

Terapia manuale

1. Please get undressed
   Si spogli per favore

2. Can you please take off your top?
   Puo togliersi il disopra?

3. Can you please take off your pants?
   Puo togliersi il pantalone?

4. Can you please take off your skirt?
   Puo togliersi la gonna?

5. Where does it hurt?
   Dove ha dei dolori?

6. Has it improved since the last treatment?
   Va meglio dal´ultima terapia?

7. Has it gotten worse?

È peggiorato?

8. Has the pain increased?

Ha più dolori di prima?

9. Has the pain gotten less?

Ha meno dolori di prima?

10. Where does it hurt now?

Dove ha adesso il dolore?

11. Stand on one leg please.

Resti su una gamba

12. Please stand on the other leg now.

Adesso su l'altra gamba

13. Stand on your heels

Si metta sui calcagni

14. Stand on your tiptoes

Resti sulle punte dei piedi

15. Sit down please
Si sieda

16. Round your back
Si metta awolto su se stesso

17. Put your chin to your chest
Avvolga la testa

18. Does it pull?
Le tira?

19. Is it painful?
Fà male?

20. Is the pain less now?
Così di meno?

21. Is the pain worse now?
Così di più?

22. Better?
Meglio?

23. Worse?

Peggio?

24. Put your head back

Alzi la testa

25. Lift your head up, look up

Alzi la testa in sù / guardi in sù

26. Put your head down, look down

In giù la testa / Guardi in giù

27. Turn your head to the left

Giri la testa a sinistra

28. Turn your head to the right

Giri la testa a destra

29. Tilt your head to the left

Pieghi la testa a sinistra

30. Tilt your head to the right

Pieghi la testa a destra

31. Relax
Rilassare

32. Do not help. I will do the movements, you relax
Non aiuti, io faccio i movimenti, si rilassi

33. Put your arms up
In alto le braccia

34. Put your right arm up
In alto il braccio destro

35. Put your right arm down
Abbassi il braccio destro

36. Put your left arm up
In alto il braccio sinistro

37. Put your left arm down
Abbassi il braccio sinistro

38. Bend your leg
Piegare la gamba

39. Extend your leg
  Stendere la gamba

40. Bend your knee
  Piegare il ginocchio

41. Extend your knee
  Stendere il ginocchio

42. Lift your leg
  Alzare la gamba

43. Lie on your back
  Si può sdraiarsi sulla schiena

44. Lie on your stomach
  Si può sdraiarsi sulla pancia

45. Lie on your right side
  Si può sdraiarsi sul´lato destro

46. Lie on your left side
  Si può sdraiarsi sul´lato sinistro

47. Put your head here, please

La testa qui per favore

48. Sit down

Si sieda

49. Please participate with ease

Faccia anche lei i movimienti insieme

50. Press against my resistance

Spinga verso la mia resistenza

51. Press harder

Spinga più forte

52. Press not so hard

Spinga più piano

53. This is an exercise to do at home

Questo è un esercizio per farlo a casa

54. Bend your legs and pull your knees to your thighs

Le gambe erette

55. Tighten your Abdomen
   Tendere la pancia

56. Squeeze your buttocks
   Tendere il sedere

57. Tense your legs
   Tendere le gambe

58. Tense your arms
   Tendere le braccia

59. Relax
   Rilasciare

60. It might hurt a little
   Puo essere che fà male un pó

61. I will show you first, then you repeat
   Io le faccio vedere, lei lo rifá

62. Do 3 sets with 10 repetitions
   Lo fá 3 volte 10

63. Do 3 sets with 15 repetitions

Lo fá 3 volte 15

64. Do 3 sets with 20 repetitions

Lo fá 3 volte 20

65. Do 3 sets with 30 repetitions

Lo fá 3 volte 30

66. Once a week

Una volta la settimana

67. Twice a week

Due volte la settimana

68. Three times a week

Tre volte la settimana

69. Once a day

Una volta al giorno

70. Twice a day

Due volte al giorno

71. Three times a day

Tre volte al giorno

72. Do the exercise in front of a mirror

Faccia questi esercizi d'avanti lo specchio

73. Sit down in front of a mirror

Si sieda d'avanti lo specchio

74. Stand in front of a mirror

Si metti in piedi d'avanti lo specchio

75. It is not supposed to hurt

Questo non deve far del male

76. This is not supposed to happen

Questo non deve succedere

PNF

Rieducazione propriocettiva

1. Lie on your back
   Si può sdraiarsi sulla schiena

2. Lie on your stomach
   Si può sdraiarsi sulla pancia

3. Lie on your right side
   Si può sdraiarsi sul lato destro

4. Lie on your left side
   Si può sdraiarsi sul lato sinistro

5. Put your head here, please
   La testa qui per favore

6. I will show you what the movement should look like
   Le faccio vedere il movimento come deve fare

7. I will do the movement, relax your arm
   Io faccio il movimento e lei lascia il braccio rilasciato

8. I will do the movement, relax your leg
   Io faccio il movimento e lei lascia la gamba rilasciata

9. Press against my resistance now
   Spinga verso la mia resistenza

10. Open your hand and extend your fingers
   Apri le dita, la mano

11. Close your hand aroung mine
   Chiuda le dita, la mano

12. Extend your arm
   Stendere il gomito

13. Bend your elbow
   Piegare il gomito

14. Put your leg up
   La gamba sù

15. Put your leg down
   La gamba giù

16. Tense your leg in this direction
   Tendere la gamba in questa direzione

17. Bend your knee
   Piegare il ginocchio

18. Extend your knee
   Stendere il ginocchio

19. Bend your hips
   Piegare i fianchi

20. Extend your hips
   Stendere i fianchi

21. Relax
   Rilassare

22. More
   Di piú

23. Less
   Di meno

24. Harder
   Piú forte

25. Softer
   Piú debole

26. Slower
   Piú piano

27. Faster
   Piú svelto

28. Press upward

    Spingere in sù

29. Press downward

    Spingere giù

30. Now in the other direction

    Adesso nell'altra direzione

31. Towards your opposite shoulder

    Direzione di fronte la spalla

32. Towards your opposite hip

    Direzione di fronte ai fianchi

33. Towards the ear

    Direzione verso l'orechio

34. Towards the nose

    Direzione verso il naso

35. Towards the window
   Direzione verso la finestra

36. Towards the door
   Direzione verso la porta

37. Towards the wall
   Direzione verso il muro

38. Towards the clock
   Direzione verso l'orologio

Mulligan

Mulligan

1. **Show me which movement causes the pain**
   Mi faccia vedere quale movimento fa male

2. **Relax**
   Si rilassi

3. **Repeat the movement once more**
   Ripeta il movimento

4. **Is it better?**
   Meglio così?

5. **Do you have pain going upstairs?**
   Ha dei dolori quando sale le scale?

6. **Do you have pain going downstairs?**
   Ha dei dolori quando scende le scale?

7. Is it better like this?

Meglio così?

8. You are not supposed to be in pain. Please say Stop if it hurts

Non deve avere dolore, se fà male mi dica "stop".

9. If the strap hurts, I can put a pad between you and the strap

Se le fà male la cinta, metto un cuscino in mezzo.

10. You can do this exercise with a towel at home

A casa puo fare questo esercizio con un asciuga mano

11. you can do this exercise at home with an elastic band

A casa può fare questo esercizio con una gomma terapotica

12. You can do this exercise at home with a stick

A casa può fare questo esercizio con un bastone

13. The ball can be purchased at a sporting goods store

Questa palla la può comprare in un negozio sportivo

14. The elastic band can be purchased at a sporting goods store

Questa gomma terapotica la puó comprare in un negozio sportivo

15. It should be red

Deve essere rosso

16. It should be green

Deve essere verde

Exercises

Esercizi

1. Bend
   Piegare

2. Extend
   Stendere

3. Flex
   Tendere

4. Relax
   Rilasciare

5. Move your buttocks backwards
   Il sedere in dietro

6. tense your abdomen / do not relax
   Tendere la pancia / lasciare teso

7. Remain like this for a few seconds, then relax
Rimanga così un paio di secondi, poi si rilasci

8. Do not move
Non ci deve essere un movimento

9. This is for your coordination
Questo e per la coordinazione

10. Do 3 sets with 10 repetitions
Lo fá 3 volte 10

11. Do 3 sets with 15 repetitions
Lo fá 3 volte 15

12. Do 3 sets with 20 repetitions
Lo fá 3 volte 20

13. Do 3 sets with 30 repetitions
Lo fá 3 volte 30

14. Take a break between the sets
Faccia delle pause durante le sedute

15. A few seconds

Un paio di secondi

16. A few minutes

Un paio di minuti

17. How many

Quanto?

18. Once a week

Una volta la settimana

19. Twice a week

Due volte la settimana

20. Three times a week

Tre volte la settimana

21. Once a day

Una volta al giorno

22. Twice a day

Due volte al giorno

23. Three times a day
Tre volte al giorno

24. Do the exercise while standing in front of a mirror
Faccia questo esercizio davanti lo specchio

25. Sit in front of the mirror
Si sieda davanti lo specchio

26. Stand in front of the mirror
In piedi davanti lo specchio

27. This is for strengthening
Questo é per rinforzare

28. Do it at home every day
Farlo ogni giorno a casa

29. Do the exercises in front of the mirror so that you can correct yourself
Faccia questi esercizi davanti lo specchio, per correggere se stesso

30. This is not supposed to happen

Questo non deve succedere

31. This is wrong

Questo é sbagliato

32. This is correct

Cosi é giusto

33. Slow

Piano

34. Slower

Più piano

35. Fast

Veloce

36. Faster

Più veloce

37. don't jerk

Non a strappi

38. Your are not supposed to be in pain during the exercise

Non deve avere dei dolori mentre fa l'esercizio

39. If you are in pain doing the exercise please stop and tell me next time you are here.

Se ha dei dolori mentre fa l'esercizio, lasci stare e melo dica la prossima volta

40. Did you do the exercises?

Ha fatto gli esercizi?

41. Did you feel any pain?

Ha avuto dei dolori mentre ha fatto l'esercizio?

42. Show me where it hurt?

Mi faccia vedere dov' era il dolore?

43. Show me how you do the exercises?

Mi faccia vedere come ha fatto l'esercizio.

44. Stand on your right leg

Stia in piedi sulla gamba destra

45. Stand on your left leg
   Stia in piedi sulla gamba sinistra

46. Stand on one leg
   Stia in piedi su una gamba

47. This is for balance
   Questo é per l'equilibrio

48. Try not to move
   Provi a non traballare

49. Try to include this exercise in your daily routine
   Questo movimento puó farlo ogni giorno

Gait Training

Rieducazione mobile

1. Stand straight
   Si metta diritto in piedi

2. Take smaller steps
   Faccia dei passi più piccoli

3. Take bigger steps
   Faccia dei passi più grande

4. Take regular steps
   Faccia dei passi regolari

5. Roll your foot from heel to toe
   Faccia scorrere il piede

6. First on your heel, roll your foot, then press your foot forward to your toes
   Prima sul calcagno, poi scorra il piede, spinga il piede avanti con il davanti del piede

7. The crutch goes on the same side as your injured leg

Questo aiuto deve andare con la gamba malata

8. Swing your arms loosely by your body

Lasci andare le braccia penzolanti per il corpo

Lymphatic drainage

Linfodrenaggio

1. **The blood pressure cannot be taken on this arm nor can blood be drawn**

   Su questo braccio non si deve misurare la pressione né fare puntura

2. **Preferably you should not get hurt**

   Cerci di non ferirsi

3. **You are not allowed to take a hot bath or lie in the sun for too long**

   Non deve fare bagno caldo né stare molto al sole

4. **If you have a painful rash, see a doctor immediately**

   Se ha un sfogo doloroso, subito del medico

5. **Put your legs up multiple times per day**

   Metta piú tempo possibile al giorno le gambe alzate

6. Put your leg up several times a day

Metta piú tempo possibile al giorno la gamba alzata

7. Put your arm up multiple times a day

Metta piú tempo possibile al giorno il braccio alzato

8. Do you have a surgical stocking?

Ha una calza antitrombose?

9. Do you have surgical stockings?

Ha delle calze antitrombose?

10. You have to wear the stocking every day

La calza la deve portare ogni giorno

11. You have to wear the stockings every day

Le calze le deve portare ogni giorno

12. You have to wear the stocking night and day

La calza la deve portare giorno e notte

13. You have to wear the stockings night and day

Le calze le deve portare giorno e notte

14. You shouldn't wear tight-fitting clothes

Non deve portare dei vestiti stretti

15. Lie on your back

Si può sdraiarsi sulla schiena

16. Lie on your stomach

Si gira sulla pancia

17. Can you lie on your stomach or would your rather sit?

Si puó sdraiare sulla pancia o meglio sedersi?

18. Sit?

Sedersi?

19. Put one leg up

Alzi la gamba

20. Put both legs up

Alzi le gambe

21. Slide a little towards me

Scivoli un pó verso di me

22. Slide to the left
Scivoli verso sinistra

23. Slide to the right
Scivoli verso destra

24. Slide up
Scivoli verso la testa

25. Slide down
Scivoli verso i piedi

26. Does it hurt?
Fà male?

27. It shouldn't hurt
Non deve far male

Electrotherapy

Elettroterapia

1. I will attach 2 electrodes

Le metto 2 elettrodi

2. I will attach 4 electrodes

Le metto 4 elettrodi

3. There is no electricity yet

Non scorre ancora corrente

4. I will increase the electricity slowly

Giro piano ad alzere la corrente

5. Tell me, as soon as you feel the electricity

Mi dica quando comincia a sentire la corrente

6. Do you feel the electricity?

Sente la corrente?

7. It should be comfortable

Deve essere gradevole

8. Is it comfortable?

É gradevole?

9. You should feel the electricity only slightly

Deve sentire la corrente leggermente

10. I will turn down the electricity until you can't feel it anymore

Ora le giro la corrente giú finché non la sente piú

11. It will take about 10 minutes

Dura ca. 10 minuti

12. It will take about 15 minutes

Dura ca 15 minuti

13. It will take about 20 minutes

Dura ca. 20 minuti

14. I will take off the electrodes once it is finished

Quando é finito vengo é gli levo gli elettrodi

15. If you have a problem, call me

Se ha dei problemi, mi chiami

16. I will be next-door

Sono quí vicino

Pelvic floor exercises

Esercizi per la Diaframma pelvico

Short

1. **The pelvic floor is the muscle between your pubic bone and your tailbone**

   Il diaframma pelvico é il muscolo frá l'osso pubico e il coccige.

2. **Its function is mainly to close the openings there**

   La sua funzione é quella di chiudere le aperture che ci si trovano

3. **It works together with you abdominal muscles and your diaphragm**

   Lavora con i muscoli addominali e con il diaframma insieme.

4. **In order to strengthen your pelvic floor you have to use these muscles as well**

   Per questo bisogna far lavorare questi muscoli per rafforzare il diaframma pelvico.

5. **Try to tense your pelvic floor, acting like have to use the bathroom but you can't go**

   Provi a tendere il diaframma pelvico come se dovesse andare in bagno ma non puó.

<u>Long</u>

1. **The pelvic floor is the muscle between ischial tuberosities, pubic and tailbone**

   Il diaframma pelvico é il muscolo che si trove trá l'osso ischio destro e sinistro, il coccige e l'osso pubico.

2. **The pelvic floor helps to control the function of urinating and bowel movement. With regular training you can prevent incontinence or lessen exiting problems**

   Il diaframma pelvico ha il compito di controllare la vostra fuori uscita di urina e feci. Per questo bisogna allenarlo regolarmente.

3. **In addition, the pelvic floor holds and supports the organs in your abdomen. That's why regular pelvic floor training works against prolapse problems**

   Il diaframma pelvico dá supporto agli organi addominali da sotto, per questo con allenamento anticipa un abbassamento degli organi.

4. **To fulfill these functions, the pelvic floor works with the abdominal muscles and the diaphragm, which is the most important respiratory muscle.**

   Per far sì che questi esercizi riecano il diaframma pelvico lavora con i muscoli addominali e il diaframma, il principale muscolo respiratorio.

5. **In order to strengthen your pelvic floor you have to use these muscles as well**

   Per questo bisogna far lavorare i muscoli per far sí che il diaframma pelvico si rafforzi

6. **Try to tighten your pelvic floor, imagining closing your vagina and anus**

   Provi a tendere il diaframma pelvico come se volesse chiudere l'ano e la sua vagina.

7. Try to tighten your pelvic floor, acting like have to use the toilet ▯but you can't go

Provi a tendere il diaframma pelvico come se devesse andare in bagno me non puó.

8. Inhale deeply. Exhale slowly tensing your abdominal muscles

Aspiri profondamente e poi respiri piano tendere la pancia

9. I will show you, and then you do it

Le faccio vedere dopo lei lo rifá.

Breathing therapy

Riabilitazione respiratoria

1. Inhale through your nose
Aspiri con il naso

2. Exhale through your mouth
Respiri con la bocca

3. I will show you, and then you do it
Le faccio vedere come deve fare, e lei lo rifá

4. Slowly
Piano

5. Slower
Più piano

6. Fast
Veloce

7. Faster
Più veloce

8. Deeply
Profondamente

9. Deeper
Più profondamente

10. Casual
Superficialmente

11. More casually
Più superficialmente

12. Inhale more into your abdomen
Respiri piu nella pancia

13. Your abdomen should expand when inhaling
La pancia deve gonfiarsi quando lei aspire

14. Put your hands on your abdomen

Mette le mani sulla pancia

15. Put your hands on your ribcage

Mette le braccia sul petto

16. Your hands should be moving on your abdomen when inhaling

Le sue mani si dovrebbero muovere dalli pancia quando lei aspire.

Useful

Utile

1. Hello
Buon giorno

2. Goodbye
Ciao

3. Please
Prego

4. Thank you
Grazie

5. Relax
Rilasci

6. Does it hurt?
Fà male?

7. Is it better now?
Meglio cosi?

8. Harder?
Più forte?

9. Yes
Si

10. No
No

11. I'm sorry, I can't understand you
Mi dispiace, ma non la capisco

English => French

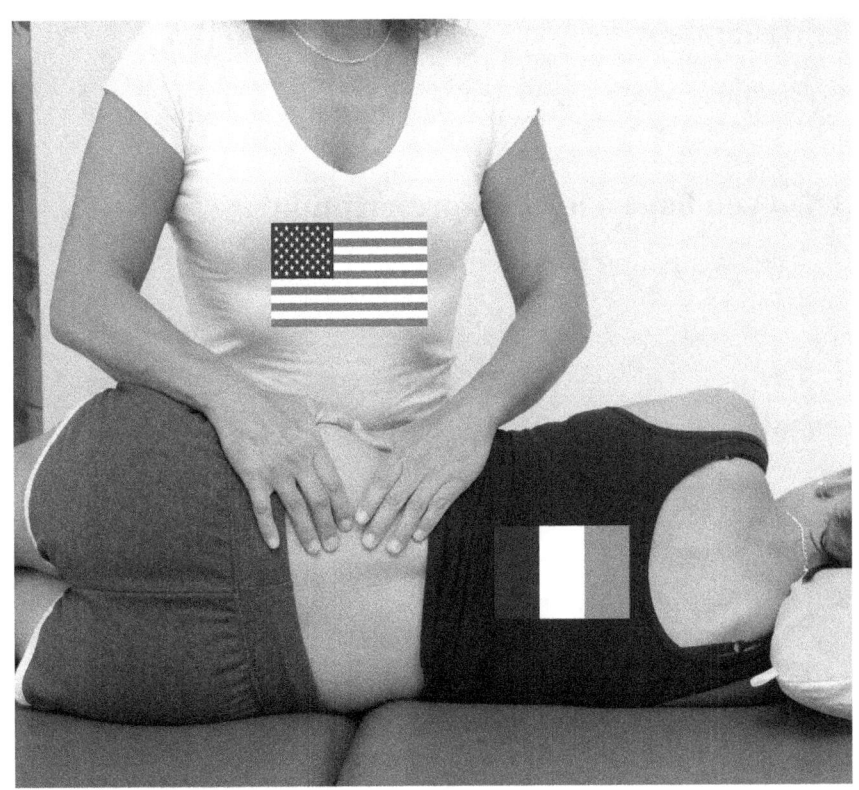

Reception

Réception

1. Hello
Bonjour

2. My name is
Je suis...

3. Do you have a doctor's prescription?
Avez-vous une ordonnance?

4. Yes
Oui

5. No
Non

6. Do you have your insurance card?
Avez-vous une carte vitale?

7. Would you please bring the insurance card next time?

Pouvez-vous apporter votre carte vitale la prochaine fois?

8. Would you please write down your phone number?

Pouvez-vous m'écrire votre numéro de téléphone, s'il vous plait?

9. There is a mistake in the prescription. You have to go back to your doctor and have him issue a new one.

Il y a une erreur sur l'ordonnance, vous devez retourner chez le medecin pour qu'il la corrige.

10. Do you have a report / X-ray / CT- images from your doctor?

Avez-vous un rapport du médecin / des radios, des tomographies?

11. Would you please bring the x-rays / the report with you next time?

Pouvez-vous amener les radios, les tomographies la prochaine fois?

12. Here are your appointments

Voici vos rendez-vous

13. If these appointments don't work for you, please let me know.

Si les rendez-vous ne vous conviennent pas, dites le moi

14. This one doesn't work?

Ça ne va pas?

15. Not on this day at all?

Pas ce jour là?

16. Rather in the morning?

Plutôt le matin

17. Rather in the afternoon?

Plutôt l'après-midi

18. Monday

Lundi

19. Tuesday
Mardi

20. Wednesday
Mercredi

21. Thursday
Jeudi

22. Friday
Vendredi

23. Saturday
Samedi

24. Sunday
Dimanche

25. I'm sorry, you are too early
Je suis désolée, vous êtes en avance

26. I'm sorry, you are too late
Je suis désolée, vous êtes en retard

27. This week won't work

Ce n'est pas possible cette semaine

28. Today doesn't work

Ce n'est pas possible aujourd´hui

29. Not before next week

A partir de la semaine prochaine

30. Not before next month

A partir du mois prochain

31. The therapist is on vacation

La / le thérapeute est en vacances

32. The therapist is ill

La / le thérapeute est malade

33. Would you like to work with a different therapist?

Voulez-vous un autre thérapeute ?

34. Yes

Oui

35. No

Non

36. Would you like to continue with the same therapist?

Voulez-vous avoir le / la même thérapeute ?

37. Would you rather wait until your therapist is back?

Voulez-vous attendre que le / la thérapeute revienne ?

38. Here is your bill.

Voici votre facture.

39. Would you like to pay now?

Voulez-vous payer maintenant ?

40. Do you want to pay cash?

Voulez-vous payer contant ?

Anamnesis

Anamnese

1. Please undress
Deshabillez vous s´il vous plait

2. Can you please take off your top ?
Pouvez-vous enlevez votre haut?

3. Can you please take off your pants?
Pouvez-vous enlever votre pantalon?

4. Can you please take off your skirt?
Pouvez-vous enlever votre jupe?

5. Are you in pain?
Avez-vous des douleurs?

6. Yes
Oui

7. **No**

   Non

8. **Show me where it hurts**

   Montrez moi où vous avez des douleurs

9. **Where does it hurt?**

   Où sont vos douleurs ?

10. **Is the pain radiating into your arm?**

    Les douleurs se diffusent-elles dans le bras?

11. **Is the pain radiating into your leg?**

    Les douleurs se diffusent-elles dans la jambe?

12. **Where does the pain radiate into?**

    Où les douleurs se diffusent-elles ?

13. **Show me**

    Montrez moi

14. Do you feel numbness?

Avez vous des zones insensibles?

15. Where?

Où?

16. Do you have paralytic symptoms?

Avez-vous des paralysies, faiblesses musculaires?

17. Do you feel formication?

Avez-vous des fourmis?

18. Where?

Où?

19. When did it start?

Depuis quand?

20. For days

Depuis plusieurs jours

21. For weeks

Depuis plusieurs semaines

22. For months

Depuis plusieurs mois

23. For years

Depuis plusieurs années

24. What does the pain feel like?

Comment est la douleur?

25. Acute

Lancinante

26. Dull

Diffuse

27. Dragging

Par élancements

28. Did the pain develop slowly?

La douleur a-t-elle commencé doucement?

29. Did the pain develop fast?

La douleur a-t-elle commencé d'un seul coup?

30. Does the pain last for a long time?

La douleur persiste-t-elle longtemps?

31. Several seconds

Plusieurs secondes

32. Several minutes

Plusieurs minutes

33. Several hours

Plusieurs heures

34. Several days

Plusieurs jours

35. Did you have an accident?
Avez-vous eu un accident?

36. Have you had treatment yet?
Avez-vous déjà recu des soins ?

37. Yes
Oui

38. No
Non

39. Do you have high blood pressure?
Faites-vous de l'hypertension?

40. Do you have diabetes?
Avez-vous le diabète?

41. Are you dizzy?
Avez-vous des vertiges?

42. Are you pregnant?

Etes-vous enceinte?

43. What month?

Depuis combien de mois?

44. Do you take pain killers?

Prenez vous des antidouleurs?

45. Do you take blood thinning medication?

Prenez vous des anticoagulants? / des médicaments?

46. Do you have problems with your thyroid?

Avez-vous des problèmes de thyroide?

47. Do you have heart problems?

Avez-vous des problèmes cardiaques?

48. Do you have a headache?

Avez-vous des maux de tête?

49. Did you have surgery?

Vous êtes vous fait opérer?

50. When did you have surgery?

Quand vous êtes vous fait opérer?

51. A few days ago

Il y a quelques jours

52. A few months ago

Il y a quelques mois

53. A few years ago

Il y a quelques années

54. You have to see a doctor.

Vous devez aller chez le médecin

55. Does it hurt when you are moving?

Avez-vous des douleurs liées à une activité / pendant une activité?

56. Do you have pain while resting?

Avez-vous des douleurs au repos?

57. When does it hurt most? When is the pain worst?

Quand les douleurs sont-elles maximales?

58. In the morning

Le matin

59. In the evening

Le soir

60. At night

La nuit

61. Always the same

Toujours pareil

62. While going up

En marchant quand ça monte

63. While going down

En marchant quand ça descend

64. Going up the stairs

En montant les escaliers

65. Going down the stairs

En descendant les escaliers

66. While sitting for a long time

Quand vous restez assis(e) longtemps?

67. After sitting for a long time

Après être resté assis(s) longtemps?

68. While doing small movements?

Lors de très petits mouvements?

69. Were you in the hospital / in rehab?

Êtes-vous allé(e) à l'hôpital/ en cure?

70. For how long?
Combien de temps ?

71. Several days
Plusieurs jours

72. Several weeks
Plusieurs semaines

73. Several months
Plusieurs mois

74. When did you get discharged from the hospital?
Quand êtes-vous sorti(e) de l'hôpital ?

75. Yesterday
Hier

76. The day before yesterday
Avant-hier

77. A few days ago

Il y a quelques jours

78. How many?

Combien ?

79. A few weeks ago

Il y a quelques semaines

80. A few months ago

Il y a quelques mois

Massage

Massage

1. Please get undressed

Vous pouvez vous déshabiller

2. Can you please take off your top?

Pouvez vous enlever votre haut?

3. Can you please take off your pants?

Pouvez vous enlever votre pantalon?

4. Can you please take off your skirt?

Pouvez vous enlever votre jupe?

5. Lie down on your back

Couchez vous sur le dos

6. Lie down on your stomach

Couchez vous sur le ventre

7. Lie down on your right side
   Couchez vous sur le côté droit

8. Lie down on your left side
   Couchez vous sur le côté gauche

9. This is for your head
   La tête ici, s´il vous plait

10. Would you like a blanket?
   Voulez-vous une couverture?

11. Are you cold?
   Avez-vous froid

12. Are you too warm?
   Avez-vous trop chaud?

13. Put your right arm down
   Mettez votre bras drois en bas

14. Put your right arm next to your head

Mettez votre bras drois en haut

15. Align your right arm alongside your body

Mettez votre bras droit le long du corps

16. Put your left arm down

Mettez votre bras gauche en bas

17. Put your left arm next to your head

Mettez votre bras gauche en haut

18. Align your left arm alongside your body

Mettez votre bras gauche le long du corps

19. Sit down please.

Asseyez-vous, s´il vous plait

20. Relax your shoulders

Détendez vos épaules

21. Please look straigt ahead

Regardez devant vous

22. Does it hurt?

Ça fait mal?

23. Do I hurt you?

Est-ce que je vous fais mal?

24. Show me where it hurts.

Montrez moi ou ça fait mal

25. Is the pressure ok?

Est-ce-que la pression est bonne / est-ce que j'appuie bien?

26. Yes?

Oui ?

27. No?

Non?

28. Harder?

Plus fort ?

29. Softer?

Moins fort?

30. Better?

C'est mieux?

31. Worse?

C'est moins bien?

Manual therapy

Thérapie manuelle

1. Please get undressed

Vous pouvez vous déshabiller

2. Can you please take off your top?

Pouvez vous enlever votre haut?

3. Can you please take off your pants?

Pouvez vous enlever votre pantalon?

4. Can you please take off your skirt?

Pouvez vous enlever votre jupe?

5. Where does it hurt?

Oú avez-vous mal / des douleurs?

6. Has it improved since the last treatment?

Est-ce que vous allez mieux depuis la dernière thérapie?

7. Has it gotten worse?

Est-ce moins bien qu'avant?

8. Has the pain increased?

Avez-vous plus de douleurs maintenant?

9. Has the pain gotten less?

Avez-vous moins de douleurs maintenant?

10. Where does it hurt now?

Où sont les douleurs maintenant / où avez-vous mal maintenant

11. Stand on one leg please.

Tenez vous sur une jambe

12. Please stand on the other leg now.

Maintenant, tenez vous sur l'autre jambe

13. Stand on your heels

Tenez vous debout seulement sur les talons

14. Stand on your tiptoes

Tenez vous debout sur la pointes des pieds

15. Sit down please

Asseyez-vous

16. Round your back

Faites le dos rond

17. Put your chin to your chest

Mettez la tête en avant / posez le menton sur votre sternum

18. Does it pull?

Ça tire?

19. Is it painful?

Ça fait mal / c'est douloureux?

20. Is the pain less now?

C'est moins douloureux comme ça?

21. Is the pain worse now?

C'est plus douloureux comme ça?

22. Better?

C'est mieux ?

23. Worse?
C'est pire?

24. Put your head back
Soulevez la tête

25. Lift your head up, look up
Regardez en l'air

26. Put your head down, look down
Regardez vers le bas / baissez la tête

27. Turn your head to the left
Tournez la tête à gauche

28. Turn your head to the right
Tournez la tête à droite

29. Tilt your head to the left
Penchez la tête à gauche

30. Tilt your head to the right
Penchez la tête à droite

31. Relax

Détendez / restez détendu(e)

32. Do not help. I will do the movements, you relax

N´essayez pas de m'aider, je fais le mouvement, vous restez détendu(e)

33. Put your arms up

Levez les bras

34. Put your right arm up

Levez le bras droit

35. Put your right arm down

Baissez le bras droit

36. Put your left arm up

Levez le bras gauche

37. Put your left arm down

Baissez le bras gauche

38. Bend your leg

Pliez la jambe

39. Extend your leg
   Tendez la jambe

40. Bend your knee
   Pliez le genou

41. Extend your knee
   Tendez le genou

42. Lift your leg
   Levez la jambe

43. Lie on your back
   Couchez vous sur le dos

44. Lie on your stomach
   Couchez vous sur le ventre

45. Lie on your right side
   Couchez vous sur le côté droit

46. Lie on your left side
   Couchez vous sur le côté gauche

47. Put your head here, please
La tête ici, s´il vous plait

48. Sit down
Asseyez vous

49. Please participate with ease
Faites le mouvement avec moi.

50. Press against my resistance
Poussez contre ma pression

51. Press harder
Poussez plus fort

52. Press not so hard
Poussez moins fort

53. This is an exercise to do at home
Ceci est un exercice à faire à la maison

54. Bend your legs and pull your knees to your thighs
Pliez les jambes et posez les pieds sous les genoux

55. Tighten your Abdomen

Contractez les muscles du ventre / faites marcher vos abdominaux

56. Squeeze your buttocks

Contractez les muscles fessiers

57. Tense your legs

Contractez les muscles des jambes

58. Tense your arms

Contractez les muscles des bras

59. Relax

Détendez vous / vos muscles

60. It might hurt a little

Il est possible que ça fasse un peu mal

61. I will show you first, then you repeat

Je vous montre, ensuite vous le faites

62. Do 3 sets with 10 repetitions

Faites trois séries à 10 répétitions

63. Do 3 sets with 15 repetitions
Faites trois séries à 15 répétitions

64. Do 3 sets with 20 repetitions
Faites trois séries à 20 répétitions

65. Do 3 sets with 30 repetitions
Faites trois séries à 30 répétitions

66. Once a week
Une fois par semaine

67. Twice a week
Deux fois par semaine

68. Three times a week
Trois fois par semaine

69. Once a day
Une fois par jour

70. Twice a day
Deux fois par jour

71. Three times a day

Trois fois par jour

72. Do the exercise in front of a mirror

Faites l'exercice devant le miroir

73. Sit down in front of a mirror

Asseyez vous devant le miroir

74. Stand in front of a mirror

Restez debout devant le miroir

75. It is not supposed to hurt

Ça ne doit pas faire mal

76. This is not supposed to happen

Ça ne doit pas arriver

PNF

Facilitation neuromusculaire par la proprioception

1. Lie on your back

   Couchez vous sur le dos

2. Lie on your stomach

   Couchez vous sur le ventre

3. Lie on your right side

   Couchez vous sur le côté droit

4. Lie on your left side

   Couchez vous sur le côté gauche

5. Put your head here, please

   La tête ici, s'il vous plait

6. I will show you what the movement should look like
Je vous montre comment faire le mouvement.

7. I will do the movement, relax your arm
Je fais le mouvement, vous laissez le bras détendu

8. I will do the movement, relax your leg
Je fais le mouvement, vous laissez la jambe détendue

9. Press against my resistance now
Maintenant, appuyez/poussez contre ma pression

10. Open your hand and extend your fingers
Ouvrez les doigts et la main

11. Close your hand aroung mine
Fermez les doigts et la main

12. Extend your arm
Tendez le coude

13. Bend your elbow
   Pliez le coude

14. Put your leg up
   Levez la jambe

15. Put your leg down
   Baissez la jambe

16. Tense your leg in this direction
   Contractez la jambe dans cette direction

17. Bend your knee
   Pliez le genou

18. Extend your knee
   Tendez le genou

19. Bend your hips
   Pliez la hanche

20. Extend your hips

Tendez la hanche

21. Relax

Détendez vous / détendez vos muscles

22. More

Plus

23. Less

Moins

24. Harder

Plus fort

25. Softer

Moins fort

26. Slower

Moins vite

27. Faster

Plus vite

28. Press upward

Appuyez, poussez vers le haut

29. Press downward

Appuyez, poussez vers le bas

30. Now in the other direction

Maintenant dans l'autre direction

31. Towards your opposite shoulder

En direction de l'épaule de l'autre côté

32. Towards your opposite hip

En direction de la hanche de l'autre côté

33. Towards the ear

Vers l'oreille

34. Towards the nose
   Vers le nez

35. Towards the window
   Vers la fenêtre

36. Towards the door
   Vers la porte

37. Towards the wall
   Vers le mur

38. Towards the clock
   Vers l'horloge

Mulligan

Mulligan

1. Show me which movement causes the pain

Montrez moi quel mouvement vous provoque des douleurs

2. Relax

Détendez vous / restez détendu

3. Repeat the movement once more

Maintenant, recommencez le mouvement.

4. Is it better?

C´est mieux?

5. Do you have pain going upstairs?

Avez vous des douleurs en montant les escaliers?

6. Do you have pain going downstairs?

Avez vous des douleurs en descandant les escaliers?

7. Is it better like this?

C'est mieux comme ça?

8. You are not supposed to be in pain. Please say Stop if it hurts

Vous ne devez pas avoir de douleurs, si ça fait mal, dites stop.

9. If the strap hurts, I can put a pad between you and the strap

Si la ceinture vous fait mal, je peux mettre un petit coussin entre vous et la ceinture.

10. You can do this exercise with a towel at home

Vous pouvez faire cet exercice à la maison avec une serviette.

11. you can do this exercise at home with an elastic band

Vous pouvez faire cet exercice à la maison avec une bande élastique.

12. You can do this exercise at home with a stick

Vous pouvez faire cet exercice à la maison avec un baton.

13. The ball can be purchased at a sporting goods store

Vous pouvez acheter la balle dans un magasin de sport.

14. The elastic band can be purchased at a sporting goods store

Vous pouvez acheter la bande élastique dans un magasin de sport.

15. It should be red

Elle doit être rouge

16. It should be green

Elle doit être verte.

Exercises

Exercices

1. Bend
Pliez

2. Extend
Tendez

3. Flex
Contractez vos muscles

4. Relax
Détendez vos muscles

5. Move your buttocks backwards
Le postérieur en arrière

6. tense your abdomen / do not relax
Contractez vos abdominaux / gardez les abdominaux contractés

7. Remain like this for a few seconds, then relax

Restez comme ça quelques secondes, ensuite détendez vos muscles

8. Do not move

Il ne doit y avoir aucun mouvement.

9. This is for your coordination

Ceci est pour la coordination

10. Do 3 sets with 10 repetitions

Faites trois séries à 10 répétitions

11. Do 3 sets with 15 repetitions

Faites trois séries à 15 répétitions

12. Do 3 sets with 20 repetitions

Faites trois séries à 20 répétitions

13. Do 3 sets with 30 repetitions

Faites trois séries à 30 répétitions

14. Take a break between the sets

Faites une pause entre les séries

15. A few seconds

Quelques secondes

16. A few minutes

Quelques minutes

17. How many

Combien

18. Once a week

Une fois par semaine

19. Twice a week

Deux fois par semaine

20. Three times a week

Trois fois par semaine

21. Once a day
   Une fois par jour

22. Twice a day
   Deux fois par jour

23. Three times a day
   Trois fois par jour

24. Do the exercise while standing in front of a mirror
   Faites l'exercice devant le miroir

25. Sit in front of the mirror
   Asseyez vous devant le miroir

26. Stand in front of the mirror
   Restez debout devant le miroir

27. This is for strengthening
   Ceci est pour la musculation

28. Do it at home every day

Faites le tous les jours à la maison

29. Do the exercises in front of the mirror so that you can correct yourself

Faites les exercices devant le miroir pour pouvoir corriger les erreurs.

30. This is not supposed to happen

Cela ne doit pas arriver

31. This is wrong

Comme ça, c'est faux

32. This is correct

Comme ça, c'est bien

33. Slow

Lentement

34. Slower

Plus lentement

35. Fast

vite

36. Faster

plus vite

37. don't jerk

Pas de mouvements brusques

38. Your are not supposed to be in pain during the exercise

Vous ne devez pas avoir de douleurs pendant des exercices.

39. If you are in pain doing the exercise please stop and tell me next time you are here.

Si vous avez des douleurs pendant les exercices, ne les faites plus et dites le moi la prochaine fois

40. Did you do the exercises?

Avez-vous fait les exercices?

41. Did you feel any pain?

Avez-vous eu des douleurs?

42. Show me where it hurt?

Montrez moi où vous avez eu des douleurs

43. Show me how you do the exercises?

Montrez moi comment vous faites l'exercice.

44. Stand on your right leg

Tenez vous debout sur la jambe droite

45. Stand on your left leg

Tenez vous debout sur la jambe gauche

46. Stand on one leg

Tenez vous debout sur une jambe

47. This is for balance

Ceci est pour l'équilibre

48. Try not to move

Essayez de ne pas tanguer

49. Try to include this exercise in your daily routine

Essayez d'intégrer ce mouvement dans votre quotidien

Gait training

Reprise de la marche

1. Stand straight
Tenez vous droit(e)

2. Take smaller steps
Faites des pas plus petits

3. Take bigger steps
Faites des pas plus grands

4. Take regular steps
Faites des pas réguliers

5. Roll your foot from heel to toe
Roulez bien le pied

6. First on your heel, roll your foot, then press your foot forward to your toes

D´abord le talon, ensuite le pied roule et se propulse en avant avec la pointe du pied

7. The crutch goes on the same side as your injured leg

Les béquilles accompagnent toujours la jambe malade

8. Swing your arms loosely by your body

Laissez les bras détendus le long du corps

Lymphatic drainage

Drainage lymphatique

1. The blood pressure cannot be taken on this arm nor can blood be drawn

On ne doit pas vous faire de prise de sang ou prendre votre tension à ce bras.

2. Preferably you should not get hurt

Vous devez faire attention à ne pas vous blesser

3. You are not allowed to take a hot bath or lie in the sun for too long

Vous ne devez pas prendre de bain brûlant ou prendre de bain de soleil

4. If you have a painful rash, see a doctor immediately

Si vous remarquez une éruption cutanée, rendez vous immédiatement chez le médecin.

5. Put your legs up multiple times per day

Surélevez les jambes souvent, plusieurs fois par jour.

6. Put your leg up several times a day

Surélevez la jambe souvent, plusieurs fois par jour.

7. Put your arm up multiple times a day

Surélevez le bras souvent, plusieurs fois par jour.

8. Do you have a surgical stocking?

Avez-vous un bas de compression?

9. Do you have surgical stockings?

Avez-vous des bas de compression?

10. You have to wear the stocking every day

Vous devez porter le bas tous les jours.

11. You have to wear the stockings every day

Vous devez porter les bas tous les jours.

12. You have to wear the stocking night and day

Vous devez porter le bas jour et nuit.

13. You have to wear the stockings night and day

Vous devez porter les bas jour et nuit.

14. You shouldn't wear tight-fitting clothes

Vous ne devez pas porter de vêtements trop serrés.

15. Lie on your back

Couchez vous sur le dos

16. Lie on your stomach

Tournez vous sur le ventre

17. Can you lie on your stomach or would your rather sit?

Pouvez-vous vous coucher sur le ventre ou préfèrez vous vous assoir?

18. Sit?

Assis(e) ?

19. Put one leg up

Pliez la jambe et posez le pied sous le genoux

20. Put both legs up

Pliez les jambes et posez les pieds sous les genoux

21. Slide a little towards me

Rapprochez vous un peu de moi

22. Slide to the left

Mettez vous un peu plus à gauche

23. Slide to the right

Mettez vous un peu plus à droite

24. Slide up

Mettez vous un peu plus haut

25. Slide down

Mettez vous un peu plus bas

26. Does it hurt?

Ça fait mal?

27. It shouldn't hurt

Ça ne doit pas faire mal

Electrotherapy

Electrothérapie

1. I will attach 2 electrodes

    Je vais poser deux électrodes

2. I will attach 4 electrodes

    Je vais poser quatre électrodes

3. There is no electricity yet

    Il n´y a pas encore de courant électrique

4. I will increase the electricity slowly

    Je monte un peu la puissance électrique

5. Tell me, as soon as you feel the electricity

    Dites le moi, dès que vous sentez l´électricité

6. Do you feel the electricity?

    Sentez-vous l´électricité?

7. It should be comfortable

Ça doit être agréable

8. Is it comfortable?

Est-ce agréable?

9. You should feel the electricity only slightly

Vous ne devez sentir qu'un léger courant électrique

10. I will turn down the electricity until you can't feel it anymore

Je baisse maintenant la puissance électrique jusqu'à ce que vous ne sentiez plus le courant.

11. It will take about 10 minutes

Cela va durer environ dix minutes

12. It will take about 15 minutes

Cela va durer environ quinze minutes

13. It will take about 20 minutes

Cela va durer environ vingt minutes

14. I will take off the electrodes once it is finished

Lorsque c´est terminé, je reviens enlever les électrodes.

15. If you have a problem, call me

S´il y a un problème, appelez moi.

16. I will be next-door

Je suis à côté

Pelvic floor exercises

Rééducation du périnée

short

1. The pelvic floor is the muscle between your pubic bone and your tailbone

Le périnée est un muscle qui se situe entre le pubis et le coccys.

2. Its function is mainly to close the openings there

Sa fonction principale est de fermer les ouvertures qui s´y trouvent.

3. It works together with you abdominal muscles and your diaphragm

Il travaille avec les muscles abdominaux et le diaphragme.

4. In order to strengthen your pelvic floor you have to use these muscles as well

C´est pour cela que ces muscles doivent aussi travailler pour remuscler le périnée.

5. Try to tense your pelvic floor, acting like have to use the bathroom but you can't go

Essayez de contracter le périnée en faisant comme si vous deviez aller aux toilettes mais que vous ne pouviez pas.

Long

1. The pelvic floor is the muscle between ischial tuberosities, pubic and tailbone

Le Périnée est le muscle situé entre les os coxaux latéraux (les os sur lesquels on s'assoit) le coccyx et le pubis.

2. The pelvic floor helps to control the function of urinating and bowel movement. With regular training you can prevent incontinence or lessen exiting problems

La fonction principale du périnée est le contrôle de la continence. Grâce à un entrainement régulier, vous pourrez éviter une incontinence ou améliorer la situation dans le cas d'une incontinence déjà présente.

3. In addition, the pelvic floor holds and supports the organs in your abdomen. That's why regular pelvic floor training works against prolapse problems

Le périnée protège et soutient les organes situés dans le bassin. C'est pour cette raison qu'un entrainement du périnée permet d'éviter une descente d'organes.

4. To fulfill these functions, the pelvic floor works with the abdominal muscles and the diaphragm, which is the most important respiratory muscle.

Afin de fonctionner correctement, le périnée travaille avec les muscles abdominaux et le diaphragme, le muscle respiratoire le plus important.

5. In order to strengthen your pelvic floor you have to use these muscles as well

C'est pour cette raison qu'il faut faire travailler ces muscles afin de remuscler le périnée.

6. Try to tighten your pelvic floor, imagining closing your vagina and anus

Essayez de contracter votre périnée en vous imaginant que vous fermer votre anus et votre vagin.

7. Try to tighten your pelvic floor, acting like have to use the toilet ▯but you can't go

Essayez de contracter votre périnéé en le contractant comme si vous aviez besoin d'aller aux toilettes mais que vous ne pouviez pas.

8. Inhale deeply. Exhale slowly tensing your abdominal muscles

Inspirez profondément, contractez votre ventre et expirez en même temps.

9. I will show you, and then you do it

Je vous montre et ensuite vous le faites.

Breathing therapy

Thérapie respiratoire

1. Inhale through your nose

Inspirez par le nez

2. Exhale through your mouth

Expirez par la bouche

3. I will show you, and then you do it

Je vous montre, ensuite vous le faites.

4. Slowly

Lentement

5. Slower

Plus lentement

6. Fast

Vite

7. Faster
Plus vite

8. Deeply
Profondément

9. Deeper
Plus profondément

10. Casual
Superficiellement

11. More casually
Moins profondément

12. Inhale more into your abdomen
Respirez plus dans le ventre

13. Your abdomen should expand when inhaling
Le ventre doit devenir plus gros lorsque vous inspirez

14. Put your hands on your abdomen

Posez vos mains sur le ventre

15. Put your hands on your ribcage

Posez vos mains sur la cage thoracique

16. Your hands should be moving on your abdomen when inhaling

Votre ventre doit faire bouger vos mains lorsque vous inspirez

Useful

Pratique

1. Hello
Bonjour

2. Goodbye
Au revoir

3. Please
S´il vous plaît

4. Thank you
Merci

5. Relax
Restez relaxé

6. Does it hurt?
C'est douloureux?

7. Is it better now?
C'est mieux comme cela?

8. Harder?
Plus fort?

9. Yes
Oui

10. No
Non

11. I'm sorry, I can't understand you
Je suis désolé, je ne comprends pas

English => German

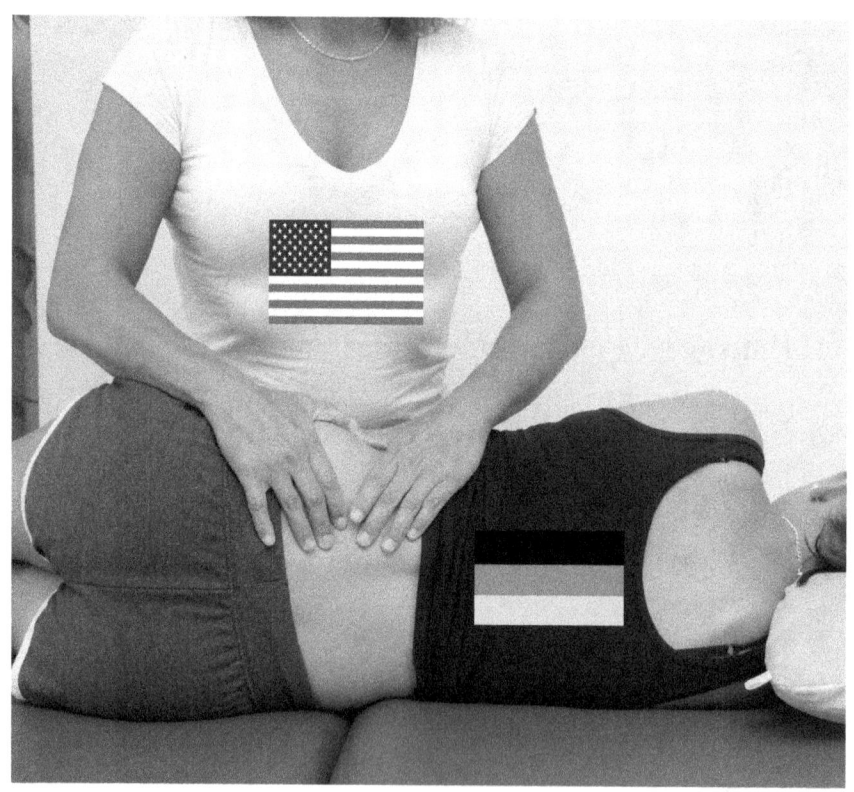

Reception

Empfang

1. Hello

Guten Tag

2. My name is

Ich heiße...

3. Do you have a doctor's prescription?

Haben Sie ein Rezept vom Arzt?

4. Yes

JA

5. No

NEIN

6. Do you have your insurance card?

Haben Sie Ihre Versicherungskarte?

7. **Would you please bring the insurance card next time?**

Können Sie das nächste mal die Karte bringen?

8. **Would you please write down your phone number?**

Können Sie mir bitte Ihre Telefonnummer aufschreiben?

9. **There is a mistake in the prescription. You have to go back to your doctor and have him issue a new one.**

Da ist ein Fehler beim Rezept, Sie müssen wieder zum Arzt damit er Ihnen ein neues Rezept gibt.

10. **Do you have a report / X-ray / CT- images from your doctor?**

Haben Sie einen Bericht / Röntgen, CT-Bilder vom Arzt?

11. **Would you please bring the x-rays / the report with you next time?**

Können Sie das nächste Mal die Bilder, den Bericht mitnehmen?

12. **Here are your appointments**

Da sind Ihre Termine

13. If these appointments don't work for you, please let me know.

Wenn die Termine für Sie nicht gehen, sagen Sie es mir.

14. This one doesn't work?

Da geht es nicht?

15. Not on this day at all?

An dem Tag nicht?

16. Rather in the morning?

Lieber Vormittags

17. Rather in the afternoon?

Lieber Nachmittags

18. Monday

Montag

19. Tuesday

Dienstag

20. Wednesday
Mittwoch

21. Thursday
Donnerstag

22. Friday
Freitag

23. Saturday
Samstag

24. Sunday
Sonntag

25. I'm sorry, you are too early
Es tut mir Leid, Sie sind zu früh

26. I'm sorry, you are too late
Es tut mir Leid, Sie sind zu spät

27. This week won't work
Diese Woche geht es nicht

28. Today doesn't work
Heute geht es nicht

29. Not before next week
Erst nächste Woche

30. Not before next month
Erst nächsten Monat

31. The therapist is on vacation
Die Therapeutin / der Therapeut ist in Urlaub

32. The therapist is ill
Die Therapeutin / der Therapeut ist krank

33. Would you like to work with a different therapist?
Wollen Sie zum anderen Therapeut ?

34. Yes
JA

35. No
NEIN

36. Would you like to continue with the same therapist?

Wollen Sie bei demselben Therapeut / derselben Therapeutin bleiben?

37. Would you rather wait until your therapist is back?

Wollen sie warten bis der Therapeut / die Therapeutin wieder da ist?

38. Here is your bill.

Hier ist Ihre Rechnung.

39. Would you like to pay now?

Wollen Sie jetzt Zahlen?

40. Do you want to pay cash?

Wollen Sie bar zahlen?

Anamnesis

Anamnese

1. Please undress

Ziehen Sie sich aus bitte

2. Can you please take off your top ?

Können Sie Ihr Oberteil ausziehen?

3. Can you please take off your pants?

Können Sie Ihre Hose ausziehen?

4. Can you please take off your skirt?

Können Sie ihren Rock ausziehen?

5. Are you in pain?

Haben Sie Schmerzen?

6. Yes

Ja

7. No

Nein

8. Show me where it hurts

Zeigen Sie mir wo Sie Schmerzen haben

9. Where does it hurt?

Wo haben Sie Schmerzen?

10. Is the pain radiating into your arm?

Strahlen Sie in den Arm aus?

11. Is the pain radiating into your leg?

Strahlen Sie in das Bein aus?

12. Where does the pain radiate into?

Bis wohin strahlen die Schmerzen?

13. Show me

Zeigen Sie es mir

14. Do you feel numbness?

Haben Sie Taubheitsgefühle?

15. Where?

Wo?

16. Do you have paralytic symptoms?

Haben Sie Lähmungserscheinungen?

17. Do you feel formication?

Haben Sie Ameisenlaufen?

18. Where?

Wo?

19. When did it start?

Seit wann?

20. For days

Seit Tagen

21. For weeks
Seit Wochen

22. For months
Seit Monaten

23. For years
Seit Jahren

24. What does the pain feel like?
Wie ist der Schmerz?

25. Acute
Stechend

26. Dull
Dumpf

27. Dragging
Ziehend

28. Did the pain develop slowly?

Ist der Schmerz langsam entstanden?

29. Did the pain develop fast?

Ist der Schmerz schnell entstanden?

30. Does the pain last for a long time?

Hält der Schmerz lange?

31. Several seconds

Mehrere Sekunden

32. Several minutes

Mehrere Minuten

33. Several hours

Mehrere Stunden

34. Several days

Mehrere Tage

35. Did you have an accident?

Hatten Sie einen Unfall?

36. Have you had treatment yet?

Sind Sie schon behandelt worden?

37. Yes

Ja

38. No

Nein

39. Do you have high blood pressure?

Haben sie Bluthochdruck?

40. Do you have diabetes?

Haben Sie Diabetis?

41. Are you dizzy?

Ist Ihnen schwindelig?

42. Are you pregnant?

Sind Sie schwanger?

43. What month?

Im wievielten Monat?

44. Do you take pain killers?

Nehmen Sie Schmerzmittel?

45. Do you take blood thinning medication?

Nehmen Sie Blutverdünnungsmedikamente / Medikamente ?

46. Do you have problems with your thyroid?

Haben Sie Probleme mit der Schilddrüse?

47. Do you have heart problems?

Haben Sie Herzprobleme?

48. Do you have a headache?

Haben Sie Kopfschmerzen?

49. Did you have surgery?

Sind Sie operiert worden?

50. When did you have surgery?

Wann sind Sie operiert worden?

51. A few days ago

Vor Tagen

52. A few months ago

Vor Monaten

53. A few years ago

Vor Jahren

54. You have to see a doctor.

Sie müssen zum Arzt gehen

55. Does it hurt when you are moving?

Haben Sie Schmerzen bei Belastung?

56. Do you have pain while resting?

Haben Sie Ruheschmerzen?

57. When does it hurt most? When is the pain worst?

Wann sind die Schmerzen am schlimmsten?

58. In the morning

Morgens

59. In the evening

Abends

60. At night

Nachts

61. Always the same

Immer gleich

62. While going up

Beim Gehen aufwärts

63. While going down

Beim Gehen abwärts

64. Going up the stairs

Beim Treppenhochsteigen

65. Going down the stairs

Beim Treppenruntersteigen

66. While sitting for a long time

Beim langen Sitzen?

67. After sitting for a long time

Nach langem Sitzen?

68. While doing small movements?

Bei kleinen Bewegungen?

69. Were you in the hospital / in rehab?

Waren Sie im Krankenhaus /Kur?

70. For how long?

Wie lange?

71. Several days

MehrereTage

72. Several weeks

Mehrere Wochen

73. Several months

Mehrere Monate

74. When did you get discharged from the hospital?

Wann sind Sie vom Krankenhaus entlassen worden?

75. Yesterday

Gestern

76. The day before yesterday

Vorgestern

77. A few days ago

Vor ein Paar Tagen

78. How many?

Wieviele ?

79. A few weeks ago

Vor ein Paar Wochen

80. A few months ago

Vor ein Paar Monaten

Massage

Massage

1. Please get undressed

Ziehen Sie sich aus bitte

2. Can you please take off your top?

Können Sie Ihr Oberteil ausziehen?

3. Can you please take off your pants?

Können Sie Ihre Hose ausziehen?

4. Can you please take off your skirt?

Können Sie ihren Rock ausziehen?

5. Lie down on your back

Legen Sie sich auf den Rücken

6. Lie down on your stomach

Legen Sie sich auf den Bauch

7. Lie down on your right side

Legen Sie sich auf die rechte Seite

8. Lie down on your left side

Legen Sie sich auf die linke Seite

9. This is for your head

Kopf hier, bitte

10. Would you like a blanket?

Wollen Sie eine Decke?

11. Are you cold?

Ist Ihnen kalt ?

12. Are you too warm?

Ist Ihnen zu warm?

13. Put your right arm down

Legen Sie den rechten Arm runter

14. Put your right arm next to your head

Legen Sie den rechten Arm hoch

15. Align your right arm alongside your body

Legen Sie den rechten Arm am Körper entlang

16. Put your left arm down

Legen Sie den linken Arm runter

17. Put your left arm next to your head

Legen Sie den linken Arm hoch

18. Align your left arm alongside your body

Legen Sie den linken Arm am Körper entlang

19. Sit down please.

Setzen Sie sich hin, bitte

20. Relax your shoulders

Schulter locker lassen

21. Please look straigt ahead

Nach vorne schauen

22. Does it hurt?

Tut es weh?

23. Do I hurt you?

Tue ich Ihnen weh?

24. Show me where it hurts.

Zeigen Sie mir wo es weh tut

25. Is the pressure ok?

Ist der Druck gut?

26. Yes?

JA ?

27. No?

NEIN?

28. Harder?

Stärker ?

29. Softer?

Schwächer ?

30. Better?

Besser?

31. Worse?

Schlechter?

Manual therapy

Manuelle Therapie

1. **Please get undressed**
   Ziehen Sie sich aus bitte

2. **Can you please take off your top?**
   Können Sie Ihr Oberteil ausziehen?

3. **Can you please take off your pants?**
   Können Sie Ihre Hose ausziehen?

4. **Can you please take off your skirt?**
   Können Sie ihren Rock ausziehen?

5. **Where does it hurt?**
   Wo haben Sie Schmerzen?

6. **Has it improved since the last treatment?**
   Ist es besser geworden seit der letzten Behandlung?

7. Has it gotten worse?

Ist es schlechter geworden?

8. Has the pain increased?

Haben Sie jetzt mehr Schmerzen?

9. Has the pain gotten less?

Haben Sie jetzt weniger Schmerzen?

10. Where does it hurt now?

Wo sind jetzt die Schmerzen?

11. Stand on one leg please.

Stehen Sie auf ein Bein

12. Please stand on the other leg now.

Jetzt auf das andere Bein stehen

13. Stand on your heels

Stehen Sie auf die Fersen

14. Stand on your tiptoes

Stehen Sie auf die Fußspitzen

15. Sit down please

Setzen Sie sich hin

16. Round your back

Machen Sie sich rund

17. Put your chin to your chest

Kopf einrollen

18. Does it pull?

Zieht es?

19. Is it painful?

Ist es schmerzhaft?

20. Is the pain less now?

So weniger ?

21. Is the pain worse now?

So mehr?

22. Better?

Besser ?

23. Worse?
schlechter?

24. Put your head back
Heben Sie den Kopf

25. Lift your head up, look up
Kopf nach oben / nach oben schauen

26. Put your head down, look down
Kopf nach unten / nach unten schauen

27. Turn your head to the left
Kopf nach links drehen

28. Turn your head to the right
Kopf nach rechts drehen

29. Tilt your head to the left
Kopf nach links neigen

30. Tilt your head to the right
Kopf nach rechts neigen

31. Relax

Locker lassen

32. Do not help. I will do the movements, you relax

Nicht helfen, ich mache die Bewegung, Sie lassen locker

33. Put your arms up

Arme hoch

34. Put your right arm up

Rechter Arm hoch

35. Put your right arm down

Rechter Arm runter

36. Put your left arm up

Linker Arm hoch

37. Put your left arm down

Linker Arm runter

38. Bend your leg

Bein beugen

39. Extend your leg

Bein strecken

40. Bend your knee

Knie beugen

41. Extend your knee

Knie strecken

42. Lift your leg

Bein heben

43. Lie on your back

Legen Sie sich auf den Rücken

44. Lie on your stomach

Legen Sie sich auf den Bauch

45. Lie on your right side

Legen Sie sich auf die rechte Seite

46. Lie on your left side

Legen Sie sich auf die linke Seite

47. Put your head here, please

Kopf hier, bitte

48. Sit down

Setzen Sie sich hin

49. Please participate with ease

Machen Sie die Bewegung leicht mit.

50. Press against my resistance

Drücken Sie gegen meinen Widerstand

51. Press harder

Drücken Sie stärker

52. Press not so hard

Drücken Sie leichter

53. This is an exercise to do at home

Das ist eine Übung für Zuhause

54. Bend your legs and pull your knees to your thighs

Beine aufstellen

55. Tighten your Abdomen

Bauch anspannen

56. Squeeze your buttocks

Po anspannen

57. Tense your legs

Beine anspannen

58. Tense your arms

Arme anspannen

59. Relax

Entspannen

60. It might hurt a little

Es kann sein, dass es ein Bißchen weh tut

61. I will show you first, then you repeat

Ich zeige es Ihnen, dann machen Sie es nach

62. Do 3 sets with 10 repetitions

Machen Sie 3 Serien à 10 Wiederholungen

63. Do 3 sets with 15 repetitions

Machen Sie 3 Serien à 15 Wiederholungen

64. Do 3 sets with 20 repetitions

Machen Sie 3 Serien à 20 Wiederholungen

65. Do 3 sets with 30 repetitions

Machen Sie 3 Serien à 30 Wiederholungen

66. Once a week

1 mal die Woche

67. Twice a week

2 mal die Woche

68. Three times a week

3 mal die Woche

69. Once a day

1 mal pro Tag

70. Twice a day

2 mal pro Tag

71. Three times a day
3 mal pro Tag

72. Do the exercise in front of a mirror
Machen Sie die Übung vor dem Spiegel

73. Sit down in front of a mirror
Sitzen Sie vor dem Spiegel

74. Stand in front of a mirror
Stehen sie vor dem Spiegel

75. It is not supposed to hurt
Das darf nicht weh tun

76. This is not supposed to happen
Das darf nicht passieren

PNF

PNF

1. Lie on your back
   Legen Sie sich auf den Rücken

2. Lie on your stomach
   Legen Sie sich auf den Bauch

3. Lie on your right side
   Legen Sie sich auf die rechte Seite

4. Lie on your left side
   Legen Sie sich auf die linke Seite

5. Put your head here, please
   Kopf hier, bitte

6. I will show you what the movement should look like
   Ich zeige Ihnen wie die Bewegung aussehen soll

7. I will do the movement, relax your arm
   Ich mache die Bewegung, Sie lassen den Arm locker

8. I will do the movement, relax your leg
   Ich mache die Bewegung, Sie lassen das Bein locker

9. Press against my resistance now
   Jetzt drücken Sie gegen meinen Widerstand

10. Open your hand and extend your fingers
   Finger, Hand aufmachen

11. Close your hand aroung mine
   Finger, Hand zumachen

12. Extend your arm
   Ellbogen strecken

13. Bend your elbow
   Ellbogen beugen

14. Put your leg up
   Bein hoch

15. Put your leg down

Bein runter

16. Tense your leg in this direction

Bein in die Richtung anspannen

17. Bend your knee

Knie beugen

18. Extend your knee

Knie strecken

19. Bend your hips

Hüfte beugen

20. Extend your hips

Hüfte strecken

21. Relax

Entspannen / locker lassen

22. More

Mehr

23. Less

Weniger

24. Harder

Stärker

25. Softer

Schwächer

26. Slower

Langsamer

27. Faster

Schneller

28. Press upward

Nach oben drücken

29. Press downward

Nach unten drücken

30. Now in the other direction

Jetzt in die andere Richtung

31. Towards your opposite shoulder

Richtung gegenüberliegende Schulter

32. Towards your opposite hip

Richtung gegenüberliegende Hüfte

33. Towards the ear

Richtung Ohr

34. Towards the nose

Richtung Nase

35. Towards the window

Richtung Fenster

36. Towards the door

Richtung Tür

37. Towards the wall

Richtung Wand

38. Towards the clock

Richtung Uhr

Mulligan

Mulligan

1. Show me which movement causes the pain
Zeigen Sie mir bei welcher Bewegung sie Schmerzen haben

2. Relax
Lassen Sie locker

3. Repeat the movement once more
Machen Sie jetzt die Bewegung noch einmal

4. Is it better?
Ist es besser?

5. Do you have pain going upstairs?
Haben Sie Schmerzen bei Treppenhochsteigen ?

6. Do you have pain going downstairs?
Haben Sie Schmerzen bei Treppenruntersteigen ?

7. Is it better like this?

Ist es besser so?

8. You are not supposed to be in pain. Please say Stop if it hurts

Sie dürfen keine Schmerzen haben, wenn es weh tut sagen Sie Stopp.

9. If the strap hurts, I can put a pad between you and the strap

Wenn der Gurt weh tut lege ich ein Polster zwischen Ihnen und dem Gurt.

10. You can do this exercise with a towel at home

Daheim können Sie diese Übung mit einem Handtuch machen

11. you can do this exercise at home with an elastic band

Daheim können Sie diese Übung mit einem Theraband machen

12. You can do this exercise at home with a stick

Daheim können Sie diese Übung mit einem Stab machen

13. The ball can be purchased at a sporting goods store

Den Ball können Sie im Sportgeschäft kaufen.

14. The elastic band can be purchased at a sporting goods store

Das Theraband können Sie im Sportgeschäft kaufen.

15. It should be red

Es soll rot sein

16. It should be green

Es soll grün sein

Exercises

Übungen

1. Bend
Beugen

2. Extend
Strecken

3. Flex
Anspannen

4. Relax
Entspannen

5. Move your buttocks backwards
Gesäß nach hinten

6. tense your abdomen / do not relax
Bauch anspannen / angespannt lassen

7. Remain like this for a few seconds, then relax

Bleiben Sie so ein Paar Sekunden, dann entspannen

8. Do not move

Es darf keine Bewegung stattfinden

9. This is for your coordination

Das ist für die Koordination

10. Do 3 sets with 10 repetitions

Machen Sie 3 Serien à 10 Wiederholungen

11. Do 3 sets with 15 repetitions

Machen Sie 3 Serien à 15 Wiederholungen

12. Do 3 sets with 20 repetitions

Machen Sie 3 Serien à 20 Wiederholungen

13. Do 3 sets with 30 repetitions

Machen Sie 3 Serien à 30 Wiederholungen

14. Take a break between the sets

Machen Sie Pause zwischen den Serien

15. A few seconds
Ein Paar Sekunden

16. A few minutes
Ein Paar Minuten

17. How many
Wieviel?

18. Once a week
1 mal die Woche

19. Twice a week
2 mal die Woche

20. Three times a week
3 mal die Woche

21. Once a day
1 mal pro Tag

22. Twice a day
2 mal pro Tag

23. Three times a day

3 mal pro Tag

24. Do the exercise while standing in front of a mirror

Machen Sie die Übung vor dem Spiegel

25. Sit in front of the mirror

Sitzen Sie vor dem Spiegel

26. Stand in front of the mirror

Stehen sie vor dem Spiegel

27. This is for strengthening

Das ist für die Kräftigung

28. Do it at home every day

Zuhause jeden Tag machen

29. Do the exercises in front of the mirror so that you can correct yourself

Machen Sie die Übungen vor dem Spiegel damit Sie sich korrigieren können

30. This is not supposed to happen
Das darf nicht passieren

31. This is wrong
Das ist falsch

32. This is correct
So ist es richtig

33. Slow
Langsam

34. Slower
Langsamer

35. Fast
Schnell

36. Faster
Schneller

37. don't jerk
Nicht ruckartig

38. Your are not supposed to be in pain during the exercise

Sie dürfen keine Schmerzen bei den Übungen haben.

39. If you are in pain doing the exercise please stop and tell me next time you are here.

Wenn Sie Schmerzen haben, während Sie die Übungen machen, lassen Sie die Übung sein und sagen es mir das nächste Mal.

40. Did you do the exercises?

Haben Sie die Übungen gemacht?

41. Did you feel any pain?

Haben Sie dabei Schmerzen gehabt?

42. Show me where it hurt?

Zeigen Sie mir wo Sie Schmerzen hatten

43. Show me how you do the exercises?

Zeigen Sie mir wie Sie die Übung machen.

44. Stand on your right leg

Stehen sie auf dem rechten Bein

45. Stand on your left leg

Stehen sie auf dem linken Bein

46. Stand on one leg

Stehen sie auf einem Bein

47. This is for balance

Das ist für das Gleichgewicht

48. Try not to move

Versuchen Sie nicht zu wackeln

49. Try to include this exercise in your daily routine

Diese Bewegung können Sie in den Alltag einbauen

Gait training

Gangschule

1. Stand straight
   Stehen Sie gerade

2. Take smaller steps
   Machen Sie kleinere Schritte

3. Take bigger steps
   Machen Sie größere Schritte

4. Take regular steps
   Machen Sie regelmäßige Schritte

5. Roll your foot from heel to toe
   Den Fuß abrollen

6. First on your heel, roll your foot, then press your foot forward to your toes

Zuerst auf Ferse, dann rollt der Fuß, dann drücken Sie den Fuß vor mit dem Vorfuß

7. The crutch goes on the same side as your injured leg

Die Gehstütze gehen mit dem kranken Bein zusammen.

8. Swing your arms loosely by your body

Arme locker am Körper pendeln lassen

Lymphatic drainage

Lymphdrainage

1. **The blood pressure cannot be taken on this arm nor can blood be drawn**

   An diesem Arm darf man kein Blutdruck messen oder Spritzen

2. **Preferably you should not get hurt**

   Sie sollen sich möglichst nicht verletzten

3. **You are not allowed to take a hot bath or lie in the sun for too long**

   Sie dürfen nicht heiß baden oder zu lange in der Sonne liegen

4. **If you have a painful rash, see a doctor immediately**

   Wenn Sie einen schmerzhaften Ausschlag haben, gehen Sie sofort zum Arzt.

5. **Put your legs up multiple times per day**

   Legen Sie oft, mehrmals pro Tag die Beine hoch

6. Put your leg up several times a day

Legen Sie oft, mehrmals pro Tag das Bein hoch

7. Put your arm up multiple times a day

Legen Sie oft, mehrmals pro Tag den Arm hoch

8. Do you have a surgical stocking?

Haben Sie einen Kompressionsstrumpf ?

9. Do you have surgical stockings?

Haben Sie Kompressionsstrümpfe?

10. You have to wear the stocking every day

Den Strumpf müssen Sie jeden Tag tragen

11. You have to wear the stockings every day

Die Strümpfe müssen Sie jeden Tag tragen

12. You have to wear the stocking night and day

Den Strumpf müssen Sie Tag und Nacht tragen

13. You have to wear the stockings night and day

Die Strümpfe müssen Sie Tag und Nacht tragen

14. You shouldn't wear tight-fitting clothes

Sie sollen keine einengende Kleidung tragen.

15. Lie on your back

Legen Sie sich auf den Rücken

16. Lie on your stomach

Drehen Sie sich auf den Bauch

17. Can you lie on your stomach or would your rather sit?

Können Sie sich auf den Bauch legen oder wollen Sie lieber sitzen?

18. Sit?

Sitzen?

19. Put one leg up

Bein aufstellen

20. Put both legs up

Beine aufstellen

21. Slide a little towards me

Ein Bisschen zu mir rutschen

22. Slide to the left

Rutschen Sie nach links

23. Slide to the right

Rutschen Sie nach rechts

24. Slide up

Rutschen Sie kopfwärts

25. Slide down

Rutschen Sie fußwärts

26. Does it hurt?

Tut es weh?

27. It shouldn't hurt

Es darf nicht weh tun

Electrotherapy

Elektrotherapie

1. I will attach 2 electrodes

Ich werde 2 Elektroden anlegen

2. I will attach 4 electrodes

Ich werde 4 Elektroden anlegen

3. There is no electricity yet

Es fließt noch kein Strom

4. I will increase the electricity slowly

Ich drehe den Strom langsam hoch

5. Tell me, as soon as you feel the electricity

Sie sagen es mir sobald Sie Strom spüren

6. Do you feel the electricity?

Spüren Sie den Strom?

7. It should be comfortable

Es soll angenehm sein

8. Is it comfortable?

Ist es angenehm?

9. You should feel the electricity only slightly

Sie sollen den Strom nur ganz leicht spüren

10. I will turn down the electricity until you can't feel it anymore

Jetzt drehe ich den Strom runter bis Sie ihn nicht mehr spüren

11. It will take about 10 minutes

Es dauert circa 10 Minuten

12. It will take about 15 minutes

Es dauert circa 15 Minuten

13. It will take about 20 minutes

Es dauert circa 20 Minuten

14. I will take off the electrodes once it is finished

Wenn es fertig ist, komme ich und mache die Elektroden weg.

15. If you have a problem, call me

Wenn Sie ein Problem haben, rufen Sie mich.

16. I will be next-door

Ich bin nebenan

pelvic floor exercises

Beckenboden Gymnastik

<u>short</u>

1. The pelvic floor is the muscle between your pubic bone and your tailbone

Der Beckenboden ist der Muskel der zwischen Schambein und Steißbein ist.

2. Its function is mainly to close the openings there

Seine Aufgabe ist hauptsächlich die Öffnungen, die sich da befinden zu schließen.

3. It works together with you abdominal muscles and your diaphragm

Er arbeitet mit den Bauchmuskeln und mit dem Zwerchfell zusammen.

4. In order to strengthen your pelvic floor you have to use these muscles as well

Deshalb muß man diese Muskeln auch mitarbeiten lassen um den Beckenboden zu kräftigen.

5. Try to tense your pelvic floor, acting like have to use the bathroom but you can't go

Versuchen Sie den Beckenboden anzuspannen indem Sie so anspannen wie wenn Sie aufs Klo müssten, es aber nicht könnten.

Long

1. The pelvic floor is the muscle between ischial tuberosities, pubic and tailbone

Der Beckenboden ist der Muskel der sich zwischen rechter und linker Sitzbeinhöcker, Steißbein und Schambein befindet. Durch regelmäßiges Training können Sie einer Inkontinenz vorbeugen oder bestehende Probleme günstig beeinflussen.

2. The pelvic floor helps to control the function of urinating and bowel movement. With regular training you can prevent incontinence or lessen exiting problems

Der Beckenboden trägt wesentlich dazu bei, dass Sie Ihren Urin- und Stuhlabgang kontrollieren können.

3. **In addition, the pelvic floor holds and supports the organs in your abdomen. That's why regular pelvic floor training works against prolapse problems**

   Weiterhin bietet der Beckenboden den inneren Bauchorganen Halt und stützt sie von unten. Daher können Sie mit einem Becken-bodentraining Senkungsbeschwerden entgegenwirken.

4. **To fulfill these functions, the pelvic floor works with the abdominal muscles and the diaphragm, which is the most important respiratory muscle.**

   Um diese Aufgaben erfüllen zu können, arbeitet der Beckenboden zusammen mit der Bauchmuskulatur und dem Zwerchfell, dem wichtigsten Atemmuskel.

5. **In order to strengthen your pelvic floor you have to use these muscles as well**

   Deshalb muß man diese Muskeln auch mitarbeiten lassen um den Beckenboden zu kräftigen.

6. **Try to tighten your pelvic floor, imagining closing your vagina and anus**

   Versuchen Sie, die Beckenbodenmuskulatur anzuspannen indem Sie sich vorstellen daß Sie Ihren After und Ihre Scheide verschließen.

7. Try to tighten your pelvic floor, acting like have to use the toilet ❑but you can't go

Versuchen Sie den Beckenboden anzuspannen indem Sie so anspannen wie wenn Sie aufs Klo müssten, es aber nicht könnten.

8. Inhale deeply. Exhale slowly tensing your abdominal muscles

Tief einatmen, beim langsamen Ausatmen Bauch anspannen.

9. I will show you, and then you do it

Ich zeige es Ihnen, dann machen Sie es nach.

Breathing therapy

Atemtherapie

1. Inhale through your nose
Atmen Sie durch die Nase ein

2. Exhale through your mouth
Atmen Sie durch den Mund aus

3. I will show you, and then you do it
Ich mache es vor, Sie machen es nach.

4. Slowly
Langsam

5. Slower
Langsamer

6. Fast
Schnell

7. Faster

Schneller

8. Deeply

Tief

9. Deeper

Tiefer

10. Casual

Oberflächig

11. More casually

Oberflächiger

12. Inhale more into your abdomen

Atmen Sie mehr in den Bauch

13. Your abdomen should expand when inhaling

Der Bauch soll dicker werden wenn Sie einatmen.

14. Put your hands on your abdomen

Legen Sie die Hände auf den Bauch

15. Put your hands on your ribcage

Legen Sie die Hände auf den Brustkorb

16. Your hands should be moving on your abdomen when inhaling

Ihre Hände sollen vom Bauch bewegt werden wenn Sie einatmen

Useful

Nützliches

1. Hello
Guten Tag

2. Goodbye
Tschüss

3. Please
Bitte

4. Thank you
Danke

5. Relax
Locker lassen

6. Does it hurt?
Tut es weh?

7. Is it better now?

Ist es besser so?

8. Harder?

Stärker?

9. Yes

Ja

10. No

Nein

11. I'm sorry, I can't understand you

Es tut mir Leid, ich verstehe Sie nicht

English => Turkish

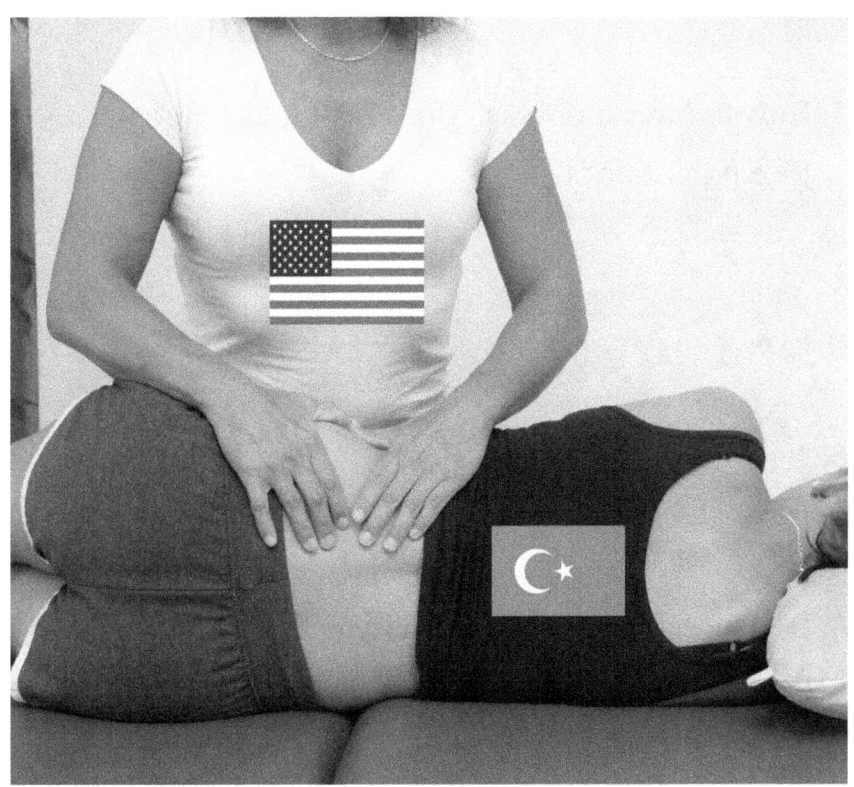

Reception

1. Hello
Iyi günler

2. My name is
Ben ...

3. Do you have a doctor's prescription?
Rezeptiniz varmı?

4. Yes
Evet

5. No
Hayır

6. Do you have your insurance card?
Sigortakartınız varmı?

7. Would you please bring the insurance card next time?
Birdahki sefere sigorta kartını getire bilirmisiniz

8. **Would you please write down your phone number?**

Telefon numaranızı yaza bilirmisiniz

9. **There is a mistake in the prescription. You have to go back to your doctor and have him issue a new one.**

Bu yalnış bir recete, doktorunuza bir başka recete isteyiniz

10. **Do you have a report / X-ray / CT- images from your doctor?**

Doktorunuzdan bir bildiri, Röntgen, CT resimleri varmı?

11. **Would you please bring the x-rays / the report with you next time?**

Birdahki sefere CT resimlerinizi getire bilirmisiniz

12. **Here are your appointments**

Bunlar sizin terminleriniz

13. **If these appointments don't work for you, please let me know.**

Terminler size uygun degilse bana bildiriniz

14. This one doesn't work?
Burada olmaz

15. Not on this day at all?
Bu günde olmaz

16. Rather in the morning?
Öğleden önce daha iyi?

17. Rather in the afternoon?
Öğleden sonra daha iyi?

18. Monday
Pazartesi

19. Tuesday
Salı

20. Wednesday
Çarşamba

21. Thursday
Perşembe

22. Friday
Cuma

23. Saturday
Cumartesi

24. Sunday
Pazar

25. I'm sorry, you are too early
Özür dilerim, ama erken geldiniz

26. I'm sorry, you are too late
Özür dilerim, ama geç geldiniz

27. This week won't work
Bu hafta olmaz

28. Today doesn't work
Bugün olmaz

29. Not before next week
En geç birdahaki hafta

30. Not before next month

En geç birdahaki ay

31. The therapist is on vacation

Terapist izinde

32. The therapist is ill

Terapist hasta

33. Would you like to work with a different therapist?

Başka bir terapisti kabul edermisiniz

34. Yes

Evet

35. No

Hayır

36. Would you like to continue with the same therapist?

Aynı terapist te kalmak istiyormusunuz?

37. Would you rather wait until your therapist is back?

Terapist gelmesini beklemek istiyormusunuz?

38. Here is your bill.

Faturanız burada

39. Would you like to pay now?

Şimdi ödemek istermisiniz

40. Do you want to pay cash?

Bar mı ödemek istiyorsunuz?

Anamnesis

1. Please undress
Lütfen üzerinizi soyunun

2. Can you please take off your top ?
Üst tarafınızı çıkarınız

3. Can you please take off your pants?
Pantolonunuzu çıkarınız

4. Can you please take off your skirt?
Eteginizi çıkarınız

5. Are you in pain?
Agrınız varmı

6. Yes
Evet

7. No
   Hayır

8. Show me where it hurts
   Nerenizde agrınız var bana gösteriniz

9. Where does it hurt?
   Nerede agrınız var?

10. Is the pain radiating into your arm?
   Agrınız kolunuza tesir ediyormu?

11. Is the pain radiating into your leg?
   Agrınız ayagınıza tesir ediyormu?

12. Where does the pain radiate into?
   Agrınız nerenize tesir ediyor?

13. Show me
   Bana gösteriniz

14. Do you feel numbness?

Uyuşukluk varmı ?

15. Where?

Nerede?

16. Do you have paralytic symptoms?

Tutukluk varmı ?

17. Do you feel formication?

Karıncılanma varmı ?

18. Where?

Nerede?

19. When did it start?

Ne zamandan beri?

20. For days

Günlerdir

21. For weeks
   Haftalardir

22. For months
   Aylardir

23. For years
   Yillardir

24. What does the pain feel like?
   Agrınız ne şekilde

25. Acute
   Igne batar şekilde

26. Dull
   Sızı şeklinde

27. Dragging
   Ceker şekilde

28. Did the pain develop slowly?

Yavaşmı Başladı agrınız?

29. Did the pain develop fast?

Hızlımı Başladı agrınız?

30. Does the pain last for a long time?

Agrınız uzun bir şüre devam ediyormu?

31. Several seconds

Saniyelerce

32. Several minutes

Dakikalarca

33. Several hours

Saatlerce

34. Several days

Günlerce

35. Did you have an accident?
Kaza geçirdinizmi?

36. Have you had treatment yet?
Müdahale edildimi

37. Yes
Evet

38. No
Hayır

39. Do you have high blood pressure?
Tansiyonunuz varmı ?

40. Do you have diabetes?
Diyabet hastalığınız varmı ?

41. Are you dizzy?
Başınız dönüyormu?

42. Are you pregnant?

Hamilemisiniz?

43. What month?

Kacıncı aydasınız?

44. Do you take pain killers?

Agrı ilaçları Kullanıyormusunuz?

45. Do you take blood thinning medication?

Kan inceltici ilaç Kullanıyormusunuz?

46. Do you have problems with your thyroid?

Kuadırınız varmı?

47. Do you have heart problems?

Kalp probleminiz varmı?

48. Do you have a headache?

Baş agrınız varmı?

49. Did you have surgery?

Ameliyal oldunuzmu?

50. When did you have surgery?

Nezaman ameliyat oldunuz?

51. A few days ago

Birkaç gün

52. A few months ago

Birkaç ay

53. A few years ago

Birkaç yıl

54. You have to see a doctor.

Doktora gitmek sorundasınız

55. Does it hurt when you are moving?

Çalışır halde agrınız varmı?

56. Do you have pain while resting?
Dinlenik bir halde agrınız varmı?

57. When does it hurt most? When is the pain worst?
Agrınız ne zaman daha fazla?

58. In the morning
Sabahları

59. In the evening
Akşamları

60. At night
Geceleri

61. Always the same
Herzaman aynı

62. While going up
Yürürken üst tarafa doğru

63. While going down

Yürürken alt tarafa doğru

64. Going up the stairs

Merdivenleri cikarken

65. Going down the stairs

Merdivenleri inerken

66. While sitting for a long time

uzun oturdugum zaman

67. After sitting for a long time

Uzun süre oturduktan sonra

68. While doing small movements?

Kisa hareketlerde

69. Were you in the hospital / in rehab?

Hasta kur ziyaretinde bulundunuzmu?

70. For how long?

Nekadar?

71. Several days

Günlerdir

72. Several weeks

Haftalardir

73. Several months

Aylardir

74. When did you get discharged from the hospital?

Nezaman hastaneden taburcu oldunuz

75. Yesterday

Dün

76. The day before yesterday

Evvelsi gün

77. A few days ago
Birkaç gün evvel

78. How many?
Kaç tane?

79. A few weeks ago
Birkaç hafta önce

80. A few months ago
Birkaç ay önce

Massage

1. **Please get undressed**
   Lütfen üzerinizi soyun

2. **Can you please take off your top?**
   Üst tarafınızı çıkarınız

3. **Can you please take off your pants?**
   Pantolonunuzu çıkarınız

4. **Can you please take off your skirt?**
   Eteginizi çıkarınız

5. **Lie down on your back**
   Sırt üstü yatınız

6. **Lie down on your stomach**
   Karnınızın üstüne yatınız

7. **Lie down on your right side**
   Sag tarafınıza yatınız

8. Lie down on your left side
Sol tarafınıza yatınız

9. This is for your head
Başınız buraya lütfen

10. Would you like a blanket?
Bastanıye istermisiniz?

11. Are you cold?
Üsuyormusunuz?

12. Are you too warm?
Sıcaklıyormusunuz?

13. Put your right arm down
Sag kolunuzu aşagıya indirin

14. Put your right arm next to your head
Sag kolunuzu yukarıya kaldırınız

15. Align your right arm alongside your body
Sag kolunuzu vucudunuza doğru tutun

16. Put your left arm down
Sol kolunuzu indirin

17. Put your left arm next to your head
Sol kolunuzu kaldırın

18. Align your left arm alongside your body
Sol kolunuzu vücudunuza doğru tutun

19. Sit down please.
Lütfen oturunuz

20. Relax your shoulders
Omuzunuzu serbest birakin

21. Please look straigt ahead
Öne doğru bakınız

22. Does it hurt?
Acıyor mu?

23. Do I hurt you?
Acıtıyormuyum?

24. Show me where it hurts.

Neresi agrıdıgını bana gösterin

25. Is the pressure ok?

Bu baskı iyimi?

26. Yes?

Evet

27. No?

Hayır

28. Harder?

Fazla?

29. Softer?

Daha az?

30. Better?

Daha iyi?

31. Worse?

Daha kötü?

Manual therapy

1. **Please get undressed**
   Lütfen üzerinizi soyun

2. **Can you please take off your top?**
   Üst tarafınızı çıkarınız

3. **Can you please take off your pants?**
   Pantolonunuzu çıkarınız

4. **Can you please take off your skirt?**
   Eteginizi çıkarınız

5. **Where does it hurt?**
   Ağrınız nerede?

6. **Has it improved since the last treatment?**
   Son müdahaleden sonra iyilesme varmı?

7. **Has it gotten worse?**
   Dahamı kötü oldu?

8. Has the pain increased?

Daha fazla agrınız varmı?

9. Has the pain gotten less?

Daha az agrınız varmı?

10. Where does it hurt now?

Şimdi agrılar nerede?

11. Stand on one leg please.

Bir ayakta durunuz

12. Please stand on the other leg now.

Şimdi diger ayagınızın üzerinde durunuz

13. Stand on your heels

Topugunuzun üzerinde durunuz

14. Stand on your tiptoes

Parmak uclarinin üzerinde durunuz

15. Sit down please

Oturunuz

16. Round your back

Kendinizi bükünüz

17. Put your chin to your chest

Başınızı eginiz

18. Does it pull?

Cekme varmı?

19. Is it painful?

Acı vericimi?

20. Is the pain less now?

Dahamı az?

21. Is the pain worse now?

Dahamı fazla?

22. Better?

Iyimi?

23. Worse?

Kötümü?

24. Put your head back

Başınızı kaldırınız

25. Lift your head up, look up

Başınızı yukarı

26. Put your head down, look down

Başınızı aşagıya

27. Turn your head to the left

Başınızı sola döndürünüz

28. Turn your head to the right

Başınızı sağa ceviriniz

29. Tilt your head to the left

Başınızı sola eğiniz

30. Tilt your head to the right

Başınızı saga eğiniz

31. Relax

Serbest bırakınız

32. Do not help. I will do the movements, you relax

Yardım etmeyiniz, ben hareketleri yapacagım, siz serbest birakın

33. Put your arms up

Kollar yukarı

34. Put your right arm up

Sag kol yukarı

35. Put your right arm down

Sag kol aşagıya

36. Put your left arm up

Sol kol yukarı

37. Put your left arm down

Sol kol aşagıya

38. Bend your leg

Bacaklarınız eginiz

39. Extend your leg

Bacaklarınız uzatınız

40. Bend your knee
  Dizinizi eginiz

41. Extend your knee
  Dizinizi uzatınız

42. Lift your leg
  Bacagınızı kaldırınız

43. Lie on your back
  Sırt üstü yatınız

44. Lie on your stomach
  Karnınızın üstüne yatınız

45. Lie on your right side
  Sag tarafınıza yatınız

46. Lie on your left side
  Sol tarafınıza yatınız

47. Put your head here, please
  Başınız buraya lütfen

48. Sit down
Oturunuz

49. Please participate with ease
Hareketleri birlikte yapınız

50. Press against my resistance
Aksi yönde hareket ediniz

51. Press harder
Daha sert hareket ediniz

52. Press not so hard
Daha hafif hareket ediniz

53. This is an exercise to do at home
Evde yapacagınız hareketler

54. Bend your legs and pull your knees to your thighs
Bacaklarınızı kaldırınız

55. Tighten your Abdomen
Karnınızı kasınız

56. Squeeze your buttocks

Kalcanızı kasınız

57. Tense your legs

Bacaklarınızı kasınız

58. Tense your arms

Kollarınızı kasınız

59. Relax

Serbest bırakın

60. It might hurt a little

Biraz acıması mümkün

61. I will show you first, then you repeat

Ben size göstereyim, siz tekrarlayın

62. Do 3 sets with 10 repetitions

3 Adet 10 defa tekrarlayın

63. Do 3 sets with 15 repetitions

3 Adet 15 defa tekrarlayın

64. Do 3 sets with 20 repetitions
3 Adet 20 defa tekrarlayın

65. Do 3 sets with 30 repetitions
3 Adet 30 defa tekrarlayın

66. Once a week
Bir defa haftada

67. Twice a week
Iki defa haftada

68. Three times a week
Üç defa haftada

69. Once a day
Günde bir defa

70. Twice a day
Günde iki defa

71. Three times a day
Günde üç defa

72. Do the exercise in front of a mirror

Hareketleri aynanın önünde yapınız

73. Sit down in front of a mirror

Aynanın önünde oturunuz

74. Stand in front of a mirror

Aynanın önünde durunuz

75. It is not supposed to hurt

Agrı hisetmemeniz gerekir

76. This is not supposed to happen

Bunun olmaması gerekir

PNF

1. **Lie on your back**
   Sırt üstü yatınız

2. **Lie on your stomach**
   Karnınızın üstüne yatınız

3. **Lie on your right side**
   Sag tarafınıza yatınız

4. **Lie on your left side**
   Sol tarafınıza yatınız

5. **Put your head here, please**
   Başınız buraya lütfen

6. **I will show you what the movement should look like**
   Hareketlerin nasıl olacağını ben size göstereyim

7. **I will do the movement, relax your arm**
   Ben hareketleri yapıyorum, siz kolunuzu gevşek tutunuz

8. I will do the movement, relax your leg

Ben hareketleri yapıyorum, siz ayağınızı gevşek tutunuz

9. Press against my resistance now

Şimdi hareketlerime karşı durun

10. Open your hand and extend your fingers

Parmakları, Eli acınız

11. Close your hand aroung mine

Parmakları, elinizi kapatınız

12. Extend your arm

Dir seginizi uzatınız

13. Bend your elbow

Dir seginizi cekiniz

14. Put your leg up

Bacagınızı kaldırınız

15. Put your leg down

Bacagınızı indiriniz

16. Tense your leg in this direction
Bacagınızı yöne göre ayarlayınız

17. Bend your knee
Dizinizi eginiz

18. Extend your knee
Dizinizi uzatın

19. Bend your hips
Kalçanızı eğin

20. Extend your hips
Kalçanız uzatınız

21. Relax
Serbest bırakın

22. More
Çok

23. Less
Az

24. Harder
Fazla?

25. Softer
Daha az?

26. Slower
Daha yavaş

27. Faster
Daha hızlı

28. Press upward
Yukarı doğru basdırınız

29. Press downward
Aşagı doğru basdırınız

30. Now in the other direction
Şimdi diger tarafa

31. Towards your opposite shoulder
Hareket karşı yöndeki omuza

32. Towards your opposite hip
   Hareket karşı yöndeki kalçaya

33. Towards the ear
   Yön kulak

34. Towards the nose
   Yön burun

35. Towards the window
   Yön Pencere

36. Towards the door
   Yön kapi

37. Towards the wall
   Yön durar

38. Towards the clock
   Yön saat

Mulligan

1. **Show me which movement causes the pain**
   Hangi harekete agrınız var

2. **Relax**
   Serbest birakınız

3. **Repeat the movement once more**
   Hareketi tekrarlayınız

4. **Is it better?**
   Dahami iyi?

5. **Do you have pain going upstairs?**
   Agrınız varmı merdüwenden cıkarsanıs ?

6. **Do you have pain going downstairs?**
   Agrınız varmı merdüwenden asaya inerken ?

7. **Is it better like this?**
   Böyle dahami iyi?

8. **You are not supposed to be in pain. Please say Stop if it hurts**

   Agrınız olmaması gerekir, acı duyarsanız "Dur" deyiniz

9. **If the strap hurts, I can put a pad between you and the strap**

   Kayış acıtıyorsa arasına singer koyayım

10. **You can do this exercise with a towel at home**

    Evde bu hareketleri havlu ile yapa bilirsiniz

11. **you can do this exercise at home with an elastic band**

    Evde bu hareketleri therabandla yapa bilirsiniz

12. **You can do this exercise at home with a stick**

    Evde bu hareketleri degnekle yapa bilirsiniz

13. **The ball can be purchased at a sporting goods store**

    Topu spor dükanindan satin alabilirsiniz

14. The elastic band can be purchased at a sporting goods store

Theraband d spor dükanindan satin alabilir

15. It should be red

Kırmızı olsun

16. It should be green

Geşi olsun

Exercises

1. Bend
Egilin

2. Extend
Uzanın

3. Flex
Kasılın

4. Relax
Serbest bırakın

5. Move your buttocks backwards
Alnınız arkaya

6. tense your abdomen / do not relax
Karnınızı kasın, kasılmış bırakın

7. Remain like this for a few seconds, then relax
Birkaç sanıye böyledurun, sonra serbest bırakın

8. Do not move
Hareket olmamak zorunda

9. This is for your coordination
Kordine için

10. Do 3 sets with 10 repetitions
3 Kere 10 adet tekrarlayın

11. Do 3 sets with 15 repetitions
3 Adet 15 defa tekrarlayın

12. Do 3 sets with 20 repetitions
3 Adet 20 defa tekrarlayın

13. Do 3 sets with 30 repetitions
3 Adet 30 defa tekrarlayın

14. Take a break between the sets
Seriler arasında mola verin

15. A few seconds
Birkaç saniye

16. A few minutes
   Birkaç dakika

17. How many
   Kaç tane?

18. Once a week
   Bir defa haftada

19. Twice a week
   Iki defa haftada

20. Three times a week
   Üç defa haftada

21. Once a day
   Günde bir defa

22. Twice a day
   Günde iki defa

23. Three times a day
   Günde üç defa

24. Do the exercise while standing in front of a mirror
Hareketleri aynanın önünde yapınız

25. Sit in front of the mirror
Aynanın önünde oturunuz

26. Stand in front of the mirror
Aynanın önünde durunuz

27. This is for strengthening
Bu güç toplamanız için

28. Do it at home every day
Evde her gün yapınız

29. Do the exercises in front of the mirror so that you can correct yourself
Hareketleri aynanın karşısında yapınız, kendiniz kontrol edebilmeniz için

30. This is not supposed to happen
Bunun olmaması gerekir

31. This is wrong
   Bu yalnış

32. This is correct
   Böyle doğru

33. Slow
   Yavaş

34. Slower
   Daha yavaş

35. Fast
   Hızlı

36. Faster
   Daha hızlı

37. don't jerk
   Acil hareket etmeyiniz

38. Your are not supposed to be in pain during the exercise
   Hareketlerde acı hissetmemeniz gerekir

39. If you are in pain doing the exercise please stop and tell me next time you are here.

Hareketleri yaparken agrı hissederseniz, yapayınız ve bana bir dahaki sefere söyleyiniz

40. Did you do the exercises?

Hareketleri yaptınızmı?

41. Did you feel any pain?

Agrı hisettinizmi?

42. Show me where it hurt?

Nerede agrınız var bana gösteriniz

43. Show me how you do the exercises?

Hareketlerinasıl yaptınız bana gösteriniz

44. Stand on your right leg

Sag ayagınızın üzerinde durunuz

45. Stand on your left leg

Sol ayagınızın üzerinde durunuz

46. Stand on one leg

Bir ayagınızın üzerinde durunuz

47. This is for balance

Bu denge için

48. Try not to move

Hareketsıs durunuz

49. Try to include this exercise in your daily routine

Bu hareketleri yaşamınızda uygulayın

Gait training

1. **Stand straight**
   Düz durunuz

2. **Take smaller steps**
   Kısa adımlar atınız

3. **Take bigger steps**
   Uzun adımlar atınız

4. **Take regular steps**
   Sık adımlar atınız

5. **Roll your foot from heel to toe**
   Ayagınızı bükünüz

6. **First on your heel, roll your foot, then press your foot forward to your toes**
   Önce topugunuzun üzerine, sonra parmaklarınızın üzerine durunuz

7. The crutch goes on the same side as your injured leg

Bastonunuz hasta ayagınızla birlikte gider

8. Swing your arms loosely by your body

Kollarınızı vucudunuzda paralel olarak sallayınız

Lymphatic drainage

1. **The blood pressure cannot be taken on this arm nor can blood be drawn**

   Bu kolda tansiyan yada igne vurunmayınız

2. **Preferably you should not get hurt**

   Mümkün oldugu kadar yaralanmayınız

3. **You are not allowed to take a hot bath or lie in the sun for too long**

   Sicak banyo yapmayınız veya güneş altinda fazla kalmayınız

4. **If you have a painful rash, see a doctor immediately**

   Aci verici bir vakkada hemen doktora gidiniz

5. **Put your legs up multiple times per day**

   Bacaklarınızı günde birkaç defa yukarı kaldırınız

6. **Put your leg up several times a day**

   Bacagınızı günde birkaç defa yukarı kaldırınız

7. **Put your arm up multiple times a day**
   Kolunuzu günde birkaç defa yukarı kaldırınız

8. **Do you have a surgical stocking?**
   Kombres corabınız varmı?

9. **Do you have surgical stockings?**
   Kombres coraplarınız varmı?

10. **You have to wear the stocking every day**
    Corabi hergün giymelisiniz

11. **You have to wear the stockings every day**
    Corapları her gün giymelisiniz

12. **You have to wear the stocking night and day**
    Corabi gece gündüz giymelisiniz

13. **You have to wear the stockings night and day**
    Corapları gece gündüz giymelisiniz

14. **You shouldn't wear tight-fitting clothes**
    Sıkı kıyafetlerden kacınınız

15. Lie on your back

Sirt üzeri yatınız

16. Lie on your stomach

Karnınızın üzerine dönünüz

17. Can you lie on your stomach or would your rather sit?

Karnınızın üzerine uzana biliyormusunuz yada oturmakmı istersiniz

18. Sit?

Oturun?

19. Put one leg up

Ayak yukarı

20. Put both legs up

Ayaklar yukarı

21. Slide a little towards me

Biraz bana doğru kayınız

22. Slide to the left
   Sol tarafa kayınız

23. Slide to the right
   Sag tarafa kayınız

24. Slide up
   Bas yukarı kayınız

25. Slide down
   Ayak aşagi kayınız

26. Does it hurt?
   Aciyormu?

27. It shouldn't hurt
   Aci hisset memeniz gerekir

Electrotherapy

1. I will attach 2 electrodes
   Iki elektrot baglayacagım

2. I will attach 4 electrodes
   Dört elektrot baglayacagım

3. There is no electricity yet
   Henüz ceyran akmamakta

4. I will increase the electricity slowly
   Ceyranı yavas yukarı cıkar tıyorum

5. Tell me, as soon as you feel the electricity
   Ceyran hissettiginiz taktirde bana bildiriniz

6. Do you feel the electricity?
   Ceyranı hissediyormusunuz

7. It should be comfortable

Iyi bir his vermesi gerekiyor

8. Is it comfortable?

Iyi bir his veriyormu?

9. You should feel the electricity only slightly

Ceyranı cok hafif bir şekilde hissetmelisiniz

10. I will turn down the electricity until you can't feel it anymore

Ceyranı şimdi acagıya indiriyorum birşey hissetmeyene kadar

11. It will take about 10 minutes

Aşagı yukarı on dakika sürer

12. It will take about 15 minutes

Aşagı yukarı onbeş dakika sürer

13. It will take about 20 minutes

Aşagı yukarı yirmi dakika sürer

14. I will take off the electrodes once it is finished

Bittiği zaman elektrotları cikarmaya gelecegim

15. If you have a problem, call me

Bir probleminiz olursa cagrın beni

16. I will be next-door

Ben yan taraftayım

Pelvic floor exercises

Short

1. **The pelvic floor is the muscle between your pubic bone and your tailbone**

   Kalça alt kası kasıkkemiği ile arasın oturma kemiğinin

2. **Its function is mainly to close the openings there**

   Onun görevi, oradaki açık olan bölümü kapatmaktır

3. **It works together with you abdominal muscles and your diaphragm**

   Karın kasları ve böleceğinizle birlikte çalışır

4. **In order to strengthen your pelvic floor you have to use these muscles as well**

   Bu yüzden bu kasları birlikte çalıştırmak gerekiyor kalça alt kasını güçlendirmek için

5. **Try to tense your pelvic floor, acting like have to use the bathroom but you can't go**

   Kalça alt kaslarınkı kasınız, tuvalete gitmeniz gerektiğini ancak yapamadığınız hisini vermesi gerekiyor

Long

1. **The pelvic floor is the muscle between ischial tuberosities, pubic and tailbone**

   Kalça alt kası, sag ve sol kuyruk kemiği, kasık kemiği ve oturma kemiğinin arasındaki kastır

2. **The pelvic floor helps to control the function of urinating and bowel movement. With regular training you can prevent incontinence or lessen exiting problems**

   Kalça alt kası, idrar ve diskiliğinizi kontrol altında tutmanıza yardımcı olar

3. **In addition, the pelvic floor holds and supports the organs in your abdomen. Thats why regular pelvic floor training works against prolapse problems**

Bunun yanında kalça alt kasığı, iç karın organlarını tutar ve alttan destekler. Bu yüzden kalça alt kas ant man çalişmalarıda sorunsuz çökmelere karşı kaya bilirsiniz

4. **To fulfill these functions, the pelvic floor works with the abdominal muscles and the diaphragm, which is the most important respiratory muscle.**

Bu görerleri yapabilmeniz için, kalça alt kası, karın kası ve böleçiinizle birlikte çalışırı en önemli nefes kaslarıdır

5. **In order to strengthen your pelvic floor you have to use these muscles as well**

Bu yüzden bu kasleri birlikte çalıştırmak gerekiyor kalça alt kasını güçlendirmek için

6. **Try to tighten your pelvic floor, imagining closing your vagina and anus**

Kalça alt kaslarınızı kasınız, vajinanızın kapandığını hissi vemesi gerekiyor

7. Try to tighten your pelvic floor, acting like have to use the toilet but you can't go

Kalça alt kaslarınız kasınız, tuvalette gitmeniz gerektiğini ancak yapamadığınızın hissini vermesi gerekiyor

8. Inhale deeply. Exhale slowly tensing your abdominal muscles

Derin nefes alın, nefes verirken karnınızı kasınız

9. I will show you, and then you do it

Ben size gösteriyorum, siz sonra tekrarlayın

Breathing therapy

1. **Inhale through your nose**
   Burundan nefes alınız

2. **Exhale through your mouth**
   Agizdan nefes veriniz

3. **I will show you, and then you do it**
   Ben yapıyorum siz tekrar ediniz

4. **Slowly**
   Yavaş

5. **Slower**
   Daha yavaş

6. **Fast**
   Hızlı

7. Faster
Daha hızlı

8. Deeply
Derinden

9. Deeper
Daha derinden

10. Casual
Gelişi güsel

11. More casually
Daha gelişi güsel

12. Inhale more into your abdomen
Karniniza hava veriniz

13. Your abdomen should expand when inhaling
Karnınız büyümeli nefes aldığınızda

14. Put your hands on your abdomen

Ellerinizi karnınızın üzerine koyunuz

15. Put your hands on your ribcage

Ellerinizi göğüsünüze koyunuz

16. Your hands should be moving on your abdomen when inhaling

Elleriniz nefes alip vermenizde hareket etmeli

Useful

1. Hello
Iyi günler

2. Goodbye
Hoşcakalınız

3. Please
Lütfen

4. Thank you
Teçekürler

5. Relax
Serbest bırakınız

6. Does it hurt?
Acı veriyormu?

7. Is it better now?
Dahami iyi?

8. Harder?
Daha hızlı?

9. Yes
Evet

10. No
Hayır

11. I'm sorry, I can't understand you
Özür dilerim sizi anliyamıyorum

Thanks

I would like to thank all those who helped me to create the Little Physio book and application.

Thanks to the translators and the proof-readers, thanks to my family and my friends who have all participated in this adventure.

Thanks to those who helped with their voice on the apps and the videos.

Special thanks to my husband who programmed the apps for android and apple and for everything else too... :)

Thank you, dear reader for having bought this book or any of my other books.

If you have enjoyed Little Physio,
please leave comments on Amazon.

I would appreciate it very much :)

Bibliography

- **Little Physio** from English into Spanish
- **Little Physio** from English into Italian
- **Little Physio** from English into French
- **Little Physio** from English into German
- **Little Physio** from English into Turkish

and

- **Big Little Physio** from English into Spanish, Italian, French, German and Turkish